Handbook of
Obstetrics & Gynecology
in Chinese Medicine

An Integrated Approach

Handbook of
Obstetrics & Gynecology
in Chinese Medicine

An Integrated Approach

Yu Jin, M.D.

TRANSLATED & EDITED BY
Chris Hakim

EASTLAND PRESS ◆ SEATTLE

Library of Congress Catalog Card Number: 97-76732
International Standard Book Number: 0-939616-28-9
Printed in the United States of America

4   6   8   10   9   7   5

Book design by Gary Niemeier

Contents

Foreword

OR OVER TEN YEARS, since I first began training foreign medical doctors both in Shanghai and abroad, I have been urged to write a book in English that would describe both the theory of traditional Chinese medicine (TCM) and its clinical applications. I did not agree to do so until 1992 when I met Chris Hakim, who was then completing an internship in TCM at Shanghai Medical University.

Countless studies have demonstrated the responsiveness of various ailments to acupuncture and herbal treatment without side effects. We are still a long way from a complete scientific explanation of the processes at work, let alone a unified model that would encompass the insights and terminologies of both Western and Chinese medical systems. But it is important to start on this path.

My initial training was in Western medicine, or biomedicine. I have since studied and practiced TCM both in clinical and research settings for almost 40 years, mostly in obstetrics and gynecology. To this day I do not think that we should try to explain TCM by any anatomical or functional system not already known to modern medicine. In the biomedical field, a virtual explosion of new knowledge and understanding has taken place over the last ten years. This has not only shed new light on the function of the human body, both in health and illness, but has also provided new mechanisms for understanding how TCM might work, and some rationales for its methods. Many studies in TCM reveal consistent histological, cellular, and molecular changes involved in conditions previously described in the traditional literature in abstract holistic terms. To cite a few examples:

- Studies on prostaglandins: changes in prostaglandins are similar to the TCM pattern of blood stasis, and are affected by herbs that invigorate the flow of blood.

- Studies on muscular tension and neurotransmitters: qi stagnancy or deficiency are usually related to the tenseness of various muscles (mostly smooth muscle), as in functional dysmenorrhea.

- Reproductive neuroendocrinology: acupuncture can change various types of central opioid levels and thus affect estrogen levels and estrogen receptors, as in acupuncture-induced ovulation.

- Reproductive endocrinology: herbs that induce ovulation act on the hypothalamic-pituitary-ovarian axis and on the adrenal glands.

The vast body of Western medical knowledge is not sufficient, however, to guide the practitioner to an accurate TCM diagnosis or treatment. For instance, postmenopausal syndrome is thought to be a problem of cooperation between the neuroendocrine immune network, the regulation of which is found at the molecular level. But herbal treatment would address things somewhere beyond that network.

Historically, TCM and Western medicine started out from opposite polar extremes. TCM evolved from the holistic and the macroscopic, while Western medical science proceeded from insights provided by specific and microscopic observations. Each now seems to be evolving towards its opposite, TCM becoming more microscopic in its approach, and Western medicine more holistic. This trend may point the way to a new era of clinical practice.

For many years attempts have been made to merge the Western and Chinese systems of medicine. In general those attempts have not been successful, probably because they were based on the assumption that there is a one-for-one correspondence between any given TCM concept and its (apparently) equivalent Western counterpart. For instance, one could make the unexamined assumption that the syndrome of blood deficiency is the same as anemia, based only on terminology. If this process of combining both systems is to have any clinical relevance, however, we must make comparisons on the basis of diagnostic and/or therapeutic similarities rather than semantics. Without a doubt, a meticulous investigator would end up with a complex patchwork of partially overlapping correspondences rather than static one-for-one equivalencies. Even if one tried to identify all diagnostic and therapeutic correspondences with perfect scientific rigor, the result would probably be one of purely academic interest.

This is not to say that these two systems of medicine are incompatible. They can enrich each other if one proceeds carefully. For the predominantly Western practitioner, this entails looking at traditional medicine within its own frame of reference, without trying to simplify it. For the TCM practitioner, an effort is required to be cognizant of established, conventional medical practice, so that his or her practice is optimally safe and effective. In summary, my view is that combining the Western and Chinese systems can be of greatest benefit if:

- a Western medical diagnosis is performed;
- a TCM diagnosis is performed to further differentiate the condition;
- a TCM treatment strategy is chosen on the basis of TCM diagnosis;
- herbs or acupuncture points are chosen within that strategy;
- TCM treatment is refined on the basis of TCM research; and
- TCM treatment is further refined on the basis of pharmacological research, or at least does not violate basic principles of therapeutic pharmacology.

In this book I have attempted to explain my ideas in terms of broad TCM diagnostic categories, easy for a beginning practitioner to understand. The care of women, including self-care, has made great advances in China since I started practicing in 1958. Diseases are arranged here in accordance with standard Western medical diagnostic categories, and then subdivided into TCM diagnostic categories.

Note on the preparation and administration of herbs

Because there is some variation in how herbal decoctions are made, I would like to outline our procedures here. Usually we use 500-600ml for each packet of herbs. The herbs are soaked for 3-6 hours. They are brought to a boil (which should take 10-15 minutes) and then kept boiling over a low heat for another 15 minutes. At this time the volume of the decoction should be 200-250ml. It is then filtered, and the filtrate taken orally after breakfast. Then another 250-300ml of water is added to the residual herbs in the pot, brought to a boil, and kept boiling over a low heat for 15 minutes. This is then filtered, with the filtrate being taken after supper. The dregs are then discarded.

Acknowledgements

I wish to give special thanks to Chris Hakim, who translated and edited the manuscript. I am impressed by his understanding of and dedication to traditional Chinese medicine. Our cooperation has been very rewarding. I am also grateful to the staff of Eastland Press, in particular John O'Connor, for his confidence, encouragement, and courtesy, which made preparation of this book a great experience.

Professor Yu Jin
Shanghai Medical University

A Methodology of Integrated Medical Diagnosis Based on Clinical Experience

TREATMENT ACCORDING TO pattern differentiation *(bian zheng shi zhi)* is the most essential part of traditional Chinese medicine. It is this process that closely integrates the various theoretical models used in traditional Chinese medicine with clinical practice. For chronic illnesses, practitioners of traditional Chinese medicine will usually differentiate the underlying pattern based on the classic eight principles *(ba gang)*, while the four levels *(si fen)* or six stages *(liu jing)* are often used to differentiate among acute diseases.

Practitioners of traditional Chinese medicine often disagree about the diagnosis in both chronic and acute cases. This is not only because traditional diagnosis is based on signs and symptoms, but also because there are a variety of diagnostic and therapeutic models used in this form of medicine. Modern biomedicine, with its laboratory and imaging studies, can often aid in resolving these issues and help us arrive at a more accurate and systematic diagnosis. For instance, traditionally, the organic cause of a symptom such as heavy uterine bleeding could not be ascertained.

Such diagnoses as carcinoma, polyp, or any anovulatory problem were unknown. With the instruments of modern biomedicine we can give a more definitive diagnosis. In addition, modern research can help us establish more standardized diagnoses for certain problems. An example of this is asymptomatic anovulation. This is a diagnosis that cannot be made from a traditional standpoint. In modern times, when trying to help women with this problem, different practitioners of traditional Chinese medicine arrive at different diagnoses. Some regard the problem as mainly involving the Spleen, others the Liver, others the qi and blood, and still others the Kidneys. Recent systematic clinical research has indicated that the problem most often relates to a deficiency of the Kidneys.

Similarly, in the treatment of acute illness, combining the diagnostic strengths of biomedicine and traditional Chinese medicine allows us to treat patients more effectively. For example, acute puerperal endometritis can be caused by different pathogens. Our methodology for approaching this disease is first to arrive at a diagnosis based on laboratory tests, then to further refine the diagnosis and determine the treatment by means of traditional-style differentiation. This principle of combining the biomedical diagnosis of a disease with the traditional Chinese diagnosis of patterns has proven to be the more effective approach to clinical management. Over the last forty years a lot of hard work has gone into integrating traditional Chinese medicine and biomedicine. We believe that this will open a new chapter in the development of both forms of medicine. The time-tested wisdom of traditional Chinese diagnosis has been reaffirmed through study and practice over these last forty years.

Integration of Biomedical Diagnosis and Traditional Chinese Pattern Differentiation

Traditionally, pattern differentiation is macroscopically based on the classical four forms of examination *(si zhen),* in which physicians use their own senses and thought processes along with a careful history from the patient and awareness of the patient's physical and emotional environment. This is a holistic view of the patient. The well-known result of this approach is that the same treatment can be applied to patients with differently-defined diseases in biomedicine, but with similar patterns according to traditional medicine; conversely, different treatments can be given to patients having the same disease in biomedicine, but presenting with different patterns in traditional medicine. In conventional biomedicine, on the other hand, a positive diagnosis can be reached by using many kinds of laboratory aids; treatment will be made according to those findings. In this process, the relation of the illness to other systems, to the whole body, or to the environment is often ignored. By contrast, in our work we emphasize the fact that we are treating a patient and not a disease. If we want to progress in our study and practice of traditional Chinese medicine, we can benefit from integrating both trains of thought: the biomedical diagnosis of disease on the one hand, and the differentiation of patterns on the other.

Let us consider the example of a patient who suffers from functional dysmenorrhea. She may have dark menstrual fluid and lower abdominal pain. Thus the main pattern is stagnant qi and blood stasis. She may also present with qi and blood deficiency, or accumulation of cold, depending on the other symptoms. From a traditional Chinese medical perspective, there is no way to investigate whether the pain is not merely functional, that is, if there is any organic basis for the pain, such as the patient's small uterus, or pelvic nodes associated with endometriosis. There may also be elevated prostaglandin $PGF_{2\alpha}$ levels in the endometrium. $PGF_{2\alpha}$ stimulates the uterus and is responsible for the hypertonic contractions which interfere with the normal rhythmic contractions, and thereby cause lower abdominal pain. Knowing this fact can help us design more effective treatments. For example, we have learned that certain substances, such as Pollen Typhae *(pu huang)* and Excrementum Trogopteri seu Pteromi *(wu ling zhi)*, which are thought to invigorate the blood in traditional Chinese medicine, biomedically are able to reduce the levels of $PGF_{2\alpha}$. In addition to dysmenorhea, endometriosis may also present with infertility due to anovulation or luteinized unruptured follicle syndrome. Lowered progesterone levels in the lower abdominal fluids can be found. In this case, the diagnosis of Kidney deficiency is warranted, in addition to the other patterns.

3

Combining both methods of diagnosis not only means providing greater insight into the disease, but also giving due consideration to the patient as an individual. This is a rule of diagnosis in traditional Chinese medicine. Let us take another example to summarize this holistic, dialectic view. In endometriosis the chief manifestations are abdominal pain, pelvic masses, infertility, high PG levels, and low immunological values in intra-abdominal fluid. According to traditional Chinese medical diagnosis, Kidney deficiency and blood stasis are the main patterns. Liver qi obstruction, stagnant heat, or injury to the Lung vessels by pathogenic fire (leading to hemoptysis) may also be present. Usually, hemoptysis is due to pathogenic fire, but when it only occurs during menstruation, treatments aimed at clearing fire (whether in the Lungs or Liver) are not helpful. Hemoptysis accompanying endometriosis is usually due to blood stasis, and the problem can only be treated effectively with herbs that eliminate blood stasis.

Blood stasis may also be seen in patients suffering from ectopic pregnancy with abdominal pain, intra-abdominal bleeding, and vaginal bleeding. In traditional Chinese medicine, blood stasis is a very broad category. The patient may have pain, tenderness, bleeding with dark clots in the menstrual blood, blood-filled cysts, and increased blood viscosity. Endometriosis can manifest as pelvic pain, tenderness, endometrial cysts, elevated blood viscosity, and other symptoms. Many other chronic diseases involve blood stasis: various types of bleeding, heart disease, chonic infections, chronic hepatitis, cirrhosis, chronic nephritis, and chronic bronchitis, all of which are accompanied by increased blood viscosity. This may be complicated by qi stagnation, qi and blood deficiency, or Intestinal excess (constipation, fever). Blood stasis again can be seen in menorrhagia accompanied by symptoms of heavy, dark menstrual blood and petechiae on the skin and tongue. Patients may also show signs and symptoms of qi or yin deficiency, or heat from deficient yin. Laboratory findings show high endometrial TXB_2 and fibrinogen degradation product levels related to high blood viscosity and deficient blood coagulation. Some patients show pallor and fatigue associated with high PGE_2 levels, resulting in hypotonia of the uterine muscle interfering with the normal rhythmic contractions. Here we have seen four different diseases—dysmenorrhea, endometriosis, ectopic pregnancy, and menorrhagia—sharing the traditional pattern of blood stasis with different manifestations: myometrial spasms, intra-abdominal bleeding, high PG levels, high blood viscosity, high fibrinogen degradation products, blood coagulation deficiency, and heavy uterine bleeding. For all four complaints, the treatment will use herbs that remove blood stasis in combination with other herbs, depending on the particular clinical requirements. Thus blood stasis can cover a very wide range of gynecological disorders: functional dysmenorrhea, ectopic pregnancy, endometriosis, adenomyosis, pelvic inflammatory disease, habitual abortion due to maternal-fetal blood-type incompatibility, and others.

Besides the fact that different biomedically-defined diseases can be encompassed within the same traditional pattern, the most important point is that the main pattern is often complicated by additional patterns which call for further differentiation of the disease into various subtypes or stages. For example, we may encounter the case of endometriosis accompanied by hemoptysis. The Womb is closely associated with the Liver and Kidneys; chronic stasis of blood may transform into fire, which then depletes the yin of the Liver and Kidneys. Fire resulting from blood stasis, as well as fire caused by Liver yin deficiency, will "burn" the blood vessels of the Lungs and cause hemoptysis. In this case, the main pattern is blood stasis in the Womb resulting in endometriosis; the secondary pattern is Liver fire resulting in hemoptysis. It is very important that the practitioner determine which pattern is the root cause of the illness, and which is a complication resulting from the main pattern.

Grasping the Essence of
Yin/Yang and Five Phase Theory

Yin, yang, and the five phases are ancient Chinese philosophical concepts which have served as the basic foundation of Chinese medicine for over two thousand years. These are abstract concepts which do not refer to concrete objects, but nonetheless are realistic and appropriate ways of thinking, analyzing, and synthesizing in traditional Chinese medicine. Approaches such as subdividing yin or yang into more subtle gradations of yin and yang, or identifying different levels of harmony between yin and yang, or the interactions among the five phases, are all helpful in leading us to look deeper and deeper into feedback and interaction among systems, tissues, cells, and molecules in the human body. No doubt new ideas and new understandings can be found by studying and applying these concepts.

For instance, when treating polycystic ovary syndrome with herbs that tonify the Kidneys, poor results were obtained in cases where blood prolactin levels were elevated. This type of patient often complains of breast engorgement and irritability, which are signs of impairment of the Liver as a result of Kidney deficiency. When herbs that quell Liver fire were added, the results improved. Many traditional Chinese medical classics and modern manuals state that the Liver and Kidneys have a common source. In modern biomedicine, disorders of the gonads or adrenals are usually diagnosed and treated in isolation, while according to five phase theory, these organs are considered part of a whole system in close interaction. For example, in Cushing's syndrome the patient's ovulation seldom receives attention. In the clinic, herbs which tonify the Kidneys are often used to induce ovulation. Those herbs were found to act on the hypothalamic-pituitary-ovarian axis and on the hypothalamic-pituitary-adrenal axis. Herbs that act on the latter also benefit the former. Herbs for post-menopausal syndrome not only treat the symptoms, but also help regulate the patient's neuroendocrine and immune systems. By contrast, estrogen replacement therapy given in menopause may reduce the activity of the immune system. This recognition of the relationship among the various Organs in traditional Chinese medicine implies an integration of the many functions and systems of the human body into a complete, interacting system. In the study of the physiological and pathological aspects of the human body, the theories of yin and yang and the five phases are gradually becoming accepted by medical scientists and clinicians. These theories are the essence of traditional Chinese medicine.

Brief Step-by-Step
Diagnostic Methodology

Diagnosing general disorders

After examining the patient according to both biomedical and traditional methodology (interrogation, inspection, auscultation, olfaction, pulse-taking, and palpation) we may then formulate the diagnosis. Chinese medicine proceeds in two steps:

1. Identify the Organs involved. The signs and symptoms may point to several systems, but one or two must play a more important role. Below is an overview of the various physiological systems and how they relate to the traditional Chinese medical concept of the Organs.

Digestion and absorption: The Stomach serves to store the food. The Spleen relates to digestion and transportation of nutrients. The Liver regulates the qi of the Stomach, and directs it downward. The Kidneys warm the Spleen and replenish the Liver.

Respiration: The Lungs are responsible for cleaning the inhaled air and for keeping the qi flowing downward. The Kidneys' role is to promote and regulate inhalation.[1]

Blood circulation: The Heart controls blood circulation. All the blood must pass through the Lungs. The Spleen keeps the blood flowing within the blood vessels. The Liver smooths the flow of qi and blood.

Skeletal and nervous system: The Kidneys determine the essence of the bone and of the bone marrow.

Metabolism: The Kidneys regulate water circulation. The Lungs contribute to the metabolism of normal (non-pathogenic) water, while the Spleen transports the water, which can transform into pathogenic dampness.

Neuropsychiatric system: Various emotional disturbances may hurt the Organs: excessive joy may overstimulate the Heart; anger can cause stag-

7

nancy in the Liver; astonishment or fear injures the Kidneys; thinking too much tires the Spleen; and sorrow depresses the Lungs.

Muscular system: The Liver is responsible for strengthening the sinews, while the Spleen nourishes the flesh.

Endocrine and immune system: The Kidneys are said to be the essence of life, while the Liver has a common source with the Kidneys (repeated in many of the medical classics). Both relate to growth and reproduction, and can thus be associated with the functions of the hypothalamus, pituitary, ovaries, adrenals, and thyroid, which also comprise the body's immuno-neuroendocrine framework.

Skin and hair: These are related to the Lungs and Kidneys.

Face: The eyes relate to the Liver, the nose to the Lungs, the ears and teeth to the Kidneys, and the mouth to the Spleen.

2. Apply the eight principles. Once the Organs that are involved in the illness have been identified, the next step is to apply the eight diagnostic principles or parameters. The diagram below sets forth a logical and convenient method to arrive at a diagnosis based on the eight principles.

First we determine whether the disease is on a superficial (exterior) or interior level. Next we must decide whether it is deficient or excessive. Finally, we look for indications of heat or cold and derive the corresponding yin or yang pattern complex.

After identifying the Organs and applying the eight principles, we will be ready to give the diagnosis. For example, in a patient suffering from amenorrhea or chronic diarrhea, the diagnosis might well be internal cold from deficiency affecting the Spleen and the Kidneys. Sometimes both an interior and exterior aspect can occur together. They may be present at the same time, as in acute enteritis: in the beginning the patient feels cold and has a floating pulse (exterior condition) and abdominal pain or diarrhea (interior condition). Or the disease may be progressing from the exterior

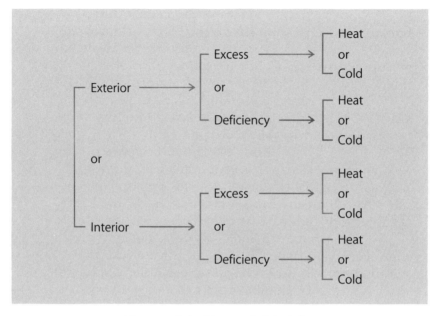

Fig. 1-1 Eight Diagnostic Principles

to the interior, as in pneumonia. An external factor may attack a patient afflicted with a chronic (that is, internal) condition. Or the disease may be said to reside *in between* the two, as with a patient suffering from alternating fever and fullness in the chest presenting with a wiry pulse and a coated tongue, in the case of malaria-like illnesses.

Similarly, excess and deficiency may sometimes appear together. In that case, it is first necessary to determine whether it is a "false" (misleading) excess or a "false" deficiency. For example, a patient suffering from dyspepsia might complain of chronic abdominal pain or distention. This would suggest stagnancy, which is a characteristic of excess. This patient could also have a pale, swollen tongue and a feeble pulse. That would indicate Spleen deficiency, wherein the qi is too weak to move the food downward. Conversely, a patient might have diarrhea and complain of poor appetite and fatigue, which is indicative of deficiency. However, if the tongue is heavily coated and the stools have a strong odor, the condition is that of food stagnancy and therefore excess. These examples reflect the

Principles	Cause(s)	Signs and Symptoms	Tongue	Pulse
exterior, excess, cold	external	chills, fever, no sweating, headache, general ache (common cold)	thin coating	floating, tense
exterior, excess, heat	external	fever, sweating, sore throat, headache (common cold)	red	floating, rapid
exterior, deficiency	qi deficiency	sweating, intolerant of wind, catches colds easily (anemia)	light, swollen	feeble
interior, excess, heat	external moving inside, or blood stasis	fever and delirium, thirst, irritability, dark urine, pain, constipation, tenderness, jaundice, coughing up yellow sputum (pneumonia, hepatitis, pelvic inflammatory disease	red or blue with thick yellow coating	rapid, forceful
interior, deficiency, heat	yin deficiency	dizziness, insomnia, bursts of irritability, palpitations, hot sensation in the five centers, thirst, dry throat, night sweats (menstrual disorders, post-menopausal syndrome)	dark, red, fissured	fine, rapid
	blood deficiency	sallow face, numbness of the fingers and toes (hypertension, stroke)	dark, red, fissured	taut
interior, deficiency, cold	qi deficiency	shortness of breath, poor appetite, abdominal distention and pain, desire for warmth, pallor, fatigue, weak voice, (chronic diarrhea, menstrual disorders, uterine prolapse	swollen, light, moist white coating	fine, weak
	yang deficiency	cold sensation, frequent and abundant urination, loose stools (functional diarrhea, amenorrhea, hypothyroidism)	swollen, light	fine, weak

Fig. 1-2 Pattern Complexes Based on Eight Diagnostic Principles

importance of the tongue and pulse in traditional diagnosis, but they also remind us to consider every factor in a case, rather than making the diagnosis based solely on the tongue and pulse.

Heat and cold may also coexist in the same patient. If someone feels cold in the lower part of the body but hot in the upper part, this is mostly a case of cold. For a common cold with fever, no sweating or thirst, but an aversion to cold, the condition is one of superficial cold, not heat. If a patient feels cold but averse to wearing warm clothing, feels thirsty, and has constipation and a rapid pulse, that patient actually suffers from a condition of heat rather than cold.

We have shown a practical approach for making a traditional Chinese medical diagnosis (Fig. 1-2). An accurate diagnosis provides the basis for formulating an effective prescription.

Weather, region, and environment

Traditional Chinese medicine recognizes that different patients suffering from the same illness may display different symptoms because of variations in weather, region, emotional state, and activity. While these principles are not mentioned explicitly in the remainder of this work, they should always be borne in mind by the conscientious practitioner. For example, in the spring the wind blows and everything rises (grows). Thus people are more vulnerable to dizziness, arthritis, and other wind-related disorders. The pulse tends to be wiry. In the summer, heat and dampness make one tired and irritable, and the pulse tends to be full. In autumn, dry weather is responsible for cough and asthma. The pulse tends to be floating. In the winter the cold makes one's face wither, and the pulse tends to sink. Also, the climate differs from region to region, and people from different regions will therefore tend to suffer from different diseases. Besides emotional disturbances, sensory perceptions may also help in diagnosis. For example, a sweet taste in the mouth may indicate Spleen deficiency. In short, a patient's condition is never to be considered independently from his or her surroundings.

Detecting ovulation

A helpful tool for the practitioner is to determine whether ovulation occurs as part of a menstrual cycle. This can be used not only for infertility, but more generally for all anovulatory disorders.

The first method, although not one-hundred percent accurate, is the basal body temperature chart. The hormonal change from follicular to luteal phase brings about a rise in body temperature of about 0.3-0.4°C (1°F), which more or less coincides with the day of ovulation, plus or minus two to four days. The patient should take her temperature every morning at the same time, before rising, and draw a temperature chart starting from the first day of menses. A normal BBT chart (Fig. 1-3) shows a fairly stable temperature for each phase, with a normal difference between them. The luteal portion of the chart should last approximately ten to fourteen days.

The second method consists of observing the ovaries using ultrasound. At the appropriate time in the cycle, a follicle can be seen rupturing to release an ovum. The corpus luteum is also visible.

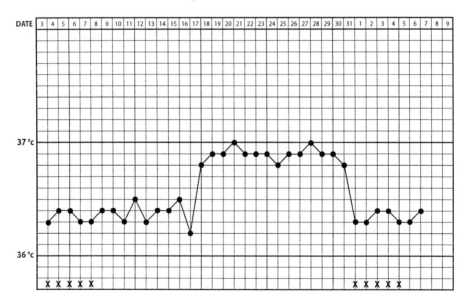

Fig. 1-3 Basal Body Temperature (BBT) Chart

This chapter dealt primarily with an approach to integrating traditional Chinese medicine with modern biomedicine based on clinical experience. This can be used by medical doctors interested in applying the insights of traditional Chinese medicine to the practice of obstetrics and gynecology. These ideas were accumulated through observation and review and are by no means a complete system of diagnostics. In the future we may look forward to a more developed approach.

Endnote

1. "Cleaning the air" is *qīng qì* in Chinese. The word *qīng* can be translated as clean, clear, or cool depending on the context.

2

Self-Care

THE INFORMATION IN this chapter is a collection of what the received tradition in Chinese medicine has to say about the subject of self-care, plus some Chinese folk wisdom. Today this folk wisdom is still observed by older Chinese women, but is often ignored by younger people. This work is the first to systematically gather all of these recommendations. A bibliography can be found at the end of the chapter.

Self-Care During Menstruation

Around the time of their periods women often experience emotional changes and are more sensitive to their environment and more vulnerable to cold. This is attributed to a mild, transient yin deficiency and a corresponding excess of yang, which are caused by the loss of blood. The following precautions may be beneficial.

Proper temperature

Warmth helps the blood circulate, too much heat causes heavy bleeding, and cold slows the flow of blood. Catching a cold, getting caught in heavy rain, coming into contact with cold water, or drinking cold beverages or herbal remedies with cold or bitter properties during menstruation—all of these factors can cause blood stasis within the Womb. This can manifest as a cessation of menstruation, oligomenorrhea, amenorrhea, or dysmenorrhea. On the other hand, pathogenic heat, very hot weather, or hot, spicy foods or herbs may invade the Womb and prolong the menses or cause menorrhagia. These factors will also affect the hypothalamic-pituitary-ovarian axis and possibly cause anovulation and infertility. It is thus necessary for a woman to pay close attention to the food, drink, and medicine she ingests, and to the temperature of the air to which she is exposed, during this part of her cycle.

Positive mood

Yin and yang are relatively imbalanced during menstruation. If a woman is unable to stay calm during this time, her mood will have a tendency to flare up, and she may become irritated, worried, or depressed at the slightest provocation, which may then cause qi stagnation, blood stasis, or the rise of fire excess. Sometimes the Kidneys and Liver are affected, leading to the appearance of menstrual disorders, amenorrhea, and other symptoms. It is therefore quite important for women to avoid quarreling and to maintain a positive attitude during menstruation.

Appropriate work and rest

Hard work, stress, strenuous exercise, and insomnia can exhaust the qi. Because qi is the commander of blood, the blood may no longer remain within the vessels or regenerate itself. Inadequate qi and blood supply to the internal organs, especially the ovaries, may cause dysfunctional uterine bleeding or amenorrhea. Women, especially pubescent girls, should thus have more rest during menstruation.

Feminine hygiene

During the menses the Womb is open and the uterine blood vessels are broken. At this time pathogenic factors may easily enter the Womb and the

Lower Burner. As a result, abnormal vaginal discharge or some menstrual disorder may be experienced because the yin channels or their collaterals have been injured. As a preventive measure, one should not douche or have sexual intercourse during vaginal bleeding. Intercourse may be harmful in two ways: first, because all the uterine blood vessels are open to the outside, leaving the woman more vulnerable to infection; and second, because it may force the flow of blood upward, rather than downward (its natural direction), and thus cause menstrual disorders. Women are also advised not to drink excessively during their periods.

Sexual intercourse should be avoided during illness or drunkenness as well, because the flow of qi in the channels and Organs might become disordered and cause menstrual problems.

All the above advice may be applied to girls as young as seven, since that is the age at which the Kidneys become stronger. When a girl reaches the age of fourteen, her essence *(jing)* reaches maturity, and her menstruation and reproductive functions follow. Keeping warm, observing a proper diet, and maintaining adequate exercise during childhood will help promote a healthy reproductive life.

Prenatal Self-Care

"Fetal education"*(tai jiao)* was mentioned in traditional Chinese medical literature a thousand years ago. Its aim was to ensure the healthy development of the fetus through its ten (lunar) months in the mother's womb. This pertains both to prenatal care as we know it, and to making a strong, healthy child. "The fetus is connected to the mother's Kidneys and is supported by the mother's qi and blood. A strong Spleen and Stomach are responsible for abundant qi and blood; thus the growth and development of the fetus mainly depend on the harmony of the mother's Kidneys, Spleen, and Stomach." Besides, the expectant mother should maintain a good mood, eat nutritious food, live a regular daily life, and avoid external pathogenic factors from the moment of conception. Both to avoid pathogenic factors, and because the Womb is connected to the Penetrating and Conception vessels, sexual activity should be avoided: it disturbs the Penetrating and Conception vessels, as well as the Kidneys, which may lead to miscarriage, premature labor, or other complications.

17

Positive mood

Harmony of the mother's qi and blood gives the fetus vitality. Adverse flow of qi and blood may jeopardize its safety and cause miscarriage. The expectant mother should therefore avoid excessive emotions such as over-joy, fright, anger, tension, depression, or sorrow, and must not become unduly worried about the sex of the child.[1]

Because of the burden of bearing a child, a woman will be weaker during pregnancy, and her mood more vulnerable. Various emotional changes may disturb the Organs or channels and cause deficiency or excess. The expectant mother should try to maintain a stable mood throughout the pregnancy, have pleasant thoughts, read, paint, enjoy music, and wear clothing that makes her feel good in order to prepare for the birth of a healthy, clever baby.

Good nutrition

Adequate diet is important during pregnancy, but it should not be too rich. Greasy, pungent, and cold foods should be avoided. One should not be partial to any particular kind of food. All these excesses can harm both the mother and the fetus. Drinking and smoking stunt the growth of the fetus.

Appropriate work and rest

Overwork injures the mother's qi and blood, while inactivity slows down the flow of qi and blood. Adequate activity is therefore suggested throughout pregnancy, not only to maintain a sufficient supply to the fetus, but also to prepare the mother for a smooth delivery. Lifting heavy things and climbing heights are forbidden.

Appropriate clothing

Loose clothing is recommended during pregnancy, to avoid obstructing the flow of qi and blood or the growth of the fetus.

Herbs contraindicated during pregnancy

The following herbs are relatively contraindicated during pregnancy because they may harm the fetus. Under special circumstances, a well-experienced physician may sometimes prescribe them.

Purgatives
Radix et Rhizoma Rhei *(da huang)*
Mirabilitum *(mang xiao)*
Semen Croton Tiglii *(ba dou)*

Blood-invigorating herbs
Semen Persicae *(tao ren)*
Flos Carthami Tinctorii *(hong hua)*
Rhizoma Sparganii Stoloniferi *(san leng)*
Rhizoma Curcumae Ezhu *(e zhu)*
Tabanus *(meng chong)*
Hirudo seu Whitmaniae *(shui zhi)*
Herba Lycopi Lucidi *(ze lan)*
Gummi Olibanum *(ru xiang)*
Radix Achyranthis Bidentatae *(niu xi)*
Spina Gleditsiae Sinensis *(zao jiao ci)*
Eupolyphaga seu Opisthoplatia *(tu bie chong)*
Lignum Sappan *(su mu)*
Herba Artemisiae Anomalae *(liu ji nu)*

Harsh expellants
Semen Pharbitidis *(qian niu zi)*
Radix Phytolaccae *(shang lu)*
Radix Euphorbiae Kansui *(gan sui)*
Radix Euphorbiae seu Knoxiae *(da ji)*
Flos Daphnes Genkwa *(yuan hua)*

Herb that expels parasites
Radix Dichroae Febrifugae *(chang shan)*

Aromatic substance that opens the orifices

Secretio Moschus *(she xiang)*

Toxic herbs

Radix Lateralis Aconiti Carmichaeli Praeparata *(fu zi)*
Radix Aconiti Kusnezoffii Praeparata *(zhi cao wu)*
Rhizoma Arisaematis *(tian nan xing)*
Rhizoma Pinelliae Ternatae *(ban xia)*
Scolopendra Subspinipes *(wu gong)*
Realgar *(xiong huang)*
Sulphur *(liu huang)*
Sal Ammoniae seu purpureum *(nao sha)*

Also note that Semen Phaseoli Radiati *(lu dou),* or mung beans, are not to be consumed during pregancy, as their cold nature can have an adverse effect on reproduction.

Postpartum Self-Care

During delivery the mother suffers a heavy loss of qi and blood from hemorrhage, injury, and exhaustion. Afterwards breast feeding further adds to her burden. According to traditional Chinese medicine, the puerperal period is defined as the four months following delivery. The first month is called "small full moon," and the remaining three are referred to as "big full moon." During the small full moon, the mother should have plenty of rest and nutrition. The precautions discussed below should also be observed. Although this section primarily deals with postpartum care, the advice also applies to women recovering from miscarriage or abortion.

Appropriate rest and activity

Except for the first twenty-four hours after delivery, the mother should try to be moderately active in order to help restore the proper flow of qi and blood and accelerate the involution of the uterus. She may gradually resume her daily work in the latter part of the big full moon. Heavy work is forbidden even after the big full moon, owing to the risk of uterine prolapse.

Appropriate clothing

During the postpartum period the mother's sweat pores are wide open, and she may perspire profusely. Her superficial resistance is lower, which means that she is more vulnerable to exogenous pathogenic influences—especially cold and dampness—which can cause stagnancy of qi and blood. The mother needs fresh air, but should not sleep in a windy area, nor wash in cold water. On the other hand, she should avoid wearing clothing that may cause her to sweat too much.

Appropriate diet

Greasy, cold, pungent, and fried foods should be avoided because of the mother's weak Spleen and Stomach. Vegetables are of value because they help prevent constipation. Foods rich in protein and vitamins are also important. Brown sugar, Arillus Euphoriae Longanae *(long yan rou)*, and Fructus Ziziphi Jujubae *(da zao)* are good for tonifying the qi and blood and speeding up the involution of the uterus. These are the traditional tonifying substances given to postpartum women.

Emotional stability

Women are often said to be more emotional than men. After delivery, blood deficiency usually is accompanied by yin deficiency and yang excess, which can become stirred up by negative emotions. Mood changes can disrupt the normal flow of qi and blood, and, in severe cases, hysteria may result.

Postpartum hygiene

Keeping the nipples clean for normal breastfeeding, changing hygienic pads regularly, and avoiding sexual activity and long baths are all important precautions to observe. It takes until the end of the "big full moon" for the Womb and the injured yin channels to recover. Sexual intercourse may resume slowly once the lochia has stopped, at the rate of once every five to nine days at first, so as not to injure the Penetrating and Conception vessels.

Perimenopausal Self-Care

Although menopause usually occurs at a definite time, typically around the age of fifty, the actual changes leading to and following this time are spread over a much longer period. Most signs and symptoms of menopause are due to a decrease in circulating estrogen. These include vasomotor irritability, vaginal dryness and irritation, a decrease in size of the breasts and uterus, and pain and stiffness in the joints. Osteoporosis may develop later. Most but not all women have vasomotor and vaginal symptoms. These phenomena remind a woman of her age and can cause a variety of emotional upsets: anxiety, depression, reduced libido, insomnia. Doctors usually prescribe estrogen replacement alone or in combination with progesterone and weak androgens. Sedatives may be of use.

According to the classical literature, once a woman reaches the age of thirty-five her yang brightness channel weakens, her essence gradually fades, and her hair begins to fall. At age forty-two the three yang channels (yang brightness, lesser yang, and greater yang) are weakened, the yin channels are affected, the face looks withered, and the hair turns gray. At age forty-nine, because of the loss of Kidney essence, the Conception and Penetrating vessels and the "heavenly dew" *(tian gui)*—which is a sexual-stimulating substance—are exhausted and menopause sets in.

The entire body, including the channels and internal Organs, begin to fade after age forty, especially the reproductive functions of the Kidneys, the bones, marrow, brain, hair, and teeth. The concept of balance is mentioned in many places in the literature, not only for physiology, pathophysiology, diagnosis, and treatment, but also for prevention. As both men and women approach the age of fifty, traditional physicians often prescribe herbal tonics based on their individual constitutions. Below are other suggestions which may enhance a woman's life around the time of menopause.

Remaining socially active whenever possible, even if one is retired, rather than staying isolated, can enhance a woman's sense of being available to others and to society. People around the same age may want to gather and organize social activities. Even if their physical bodies are not as strong as those of younger people, their ability to ponder problems is more efficient and mature.

A menopausal woman may want to rearrange her lifestyle to be more calm and gentle, giving more time to her family, friends, and relatives. She might reorganize her schedule to go to bed early, get up early, avoid excesses, and choose one or two recreational activities such as music, chess, painting, calligraphy, reading, stamp collecting, fishing, growing flowers, or raising pets. Daily exercise based on individual ability is strongly advised. Qi Gong, Tai Ji, or self-massage nearly always produces positive effects on one's health and spirit. While engaged in this kind of exercise, one should remain calm internally and cultivate a sense of harmony with the external environment, breathe in deeply, and become exposed to sunlight.

Menopausal women should have plenty of fresh vegetables and fluids, digestible foods, and plenty of water and fiber in order to enhance digestion and bowel function. Meat, fatty or spicy foods, cigarettes, heavy tea, and alcohol should be reduced or avoided. Women should be mindful of the seasonal and weather changes when selecting their clothing. Finally, they should not become nervous whenever health problems develop, but seek appropriate help, rely on their physician's advice, and avail themselves of routine health-screening procedures.

Bibliography

Annonymous, *Yellow Emperor's Inner Classic (Huang di nei jing)*, c. 200 B.C.

Chen Zi-Ming, *Compendium of Fine Formulas for Women (Fu ren liang fang da quan)*, 1237.

Fu Shan, *Fu Qing-Zhu's Obstetrics and Gynecology (Fu Qing-Zhu nu ke)*, 1827.

Wu Qian et al., *Golden Mirror of Medicine (Yin zong jin jian)*, 1742.

Wu Zhi-Wang, *Compendium of Therapy for Women's Diseases (Ji yin gang mu)*, 1620.

Zhu Zhen-Heng, *Teachings of [Zhu] Dan-Xi (Dan-Xi xin fa)*, 1481.

Endnote

1. In feudal China, women were looked down upon, thus expectant mothers were under a lot of pressure from their relatives to bear a son rather than a daughter.

Disorders of the Vulva

Vulvar Dystrophy

VULVAR DYSTROPHIES REPRESENT a spectrum of atrophic and hypertrophic changes caused by chronic stimulation, leading to the "white lesions" of the vulva.

Hypertrophic changes may be caused by chronic vulvovaginal infections or other stimulation resulting in benign epithelial thickening and hyperkeratosis. These lesions do not have a uniform, characteristic microscopic appearance. It is therefore necessary to perform periodic biopsies to rule out malignancy.

Atrophic changes result from a decrease in endogenous estrogen in older women. Chief symptoms include dysuria, dyspareunia, and pruritus.

Conventional medical management of both types of lesions involves removing the causative factor, plus local treatment with creams containing estrogens, corticosteroids, or testosterone. Recently, laser treatment has been introduced. If dysplasia or malignancy is detected, appropriate therapy should be given as soon as possible.

In traditional Chinese medicine, vulvar dystrophy is differentiated as either vulvar deficiency (*yin shi*) or vulvar pruritus (*yin yang*). The Liver and Kidney channels run through the vulva, and the Kidneys are said to "open" into the vulva and anus. Kidney and Liver yin deficiency are responsible for pathogenic heat and dryness in the vulva, producing heat, itching, and dampness. The Spleen is also affected by the Liver in accordance with the five-phase relationship of "wood controlling earth." Thus, in chronic cases, qi and blood are injured and qi stagnancy and blood stasis result.

Herbal treatment

Vulvar Dystrophy Formula 1

If there is no sign of deficiency of the viscera, the formula below is used as a fumigation and sitz bath.

Fructus Cnidii Monnieri *(she chuang zi)* 30g
Alumen *(ming fan)* 12g
Radix Sophorae Flavescentis *(ku shen)* 12g
Radix Stemonae *(bai bu)* 12g
Cortex Ailanthi Altissimae *(chun pi)* 12g
Pericarpium Zanthoxyli Bungeani *(chuan jiao)* 12g

METHOD: Boil in two liters of water for twenty minutes. Expose the vulva to the fumes until the decoction is just warm, then use as a sitz bath.

ANALYSIS OF FORMULA: Fructus Cnidii Monnieri *(she chuang zi)* tonifies the Kidneys, dries dampness, and relieves itching. In animal experiments and in clinical practice, endocrine and immune activity has been shown. It also inhibits the growth of trichomonas in vitro. Alumen *(ming fan)*, Radix Sophorae Flavescentis *(ku shen)*, and Cortex Ailanthi Altissimae *(chun pi)* all clear pathogenic heat, dry dampness, and have bactericidal activity. In addition, Cortex Ailanthi Altissimae *(chun pi)* alleviates leukorrhea. Pericarpium Zanthoxyli Bungeani *(chuan jiao)* has warm properties which balance the cold properties of the other herbs. It also acts as an antiviral, bactericidal, and fungicidal agent.

Vulvar Dystrophy Formula 2

This formula is used when there is deficiency of the Liver and Kidneys. It is prepared as a decoction, sometimes in combination with the fumigation and sitz bath described above.

Herba Epimedii *(yin yang huo)* 12g
Rhizoma Polygonati *(huang jing)* 12g
Radix Morindae Officinalis *(ba ji tian)* 12g
Fructus Ligustri Lucidi *(nu zhen zi)* 12g
Semen Astragali *(sha yuan ji li)* 9g
Radix Angelicae Sinensis *(dang gui)* 9g
Cortex Moutan Radicis *(mu dan pi)* 6g
Radix Paeoniae Rubrae *(chi shao)* 12g
Radix et Caulis Jixueteng *(ji xue teng)* 12g
Periostracum Cicadae *(chan tui)* 6g
Herba Menthae Haplocalycis *(bo he)* 1.5g

ANALYSIS OF FORMULA: Herba Epimedii *(yin yang huo)*, Radix Morindae Officinalis *(ba ji tian)*, and Semen Astragali *(sha yuan ji li)* are used to tonify the Liver and Kidneys. Fructus Ligustri Lucidi *(nu zhen zi)* and Rhizoma Polygonati *(huang jing)* not only replenish the yin of the Liver, Kidneys, and Spleen, but also moderate the pungent and dry qualities of Herba Epimedii *(yin yang huo)*. Radix Angelicae Sinensis *(dang gui)*, Radix Paeoniae Rubrae *(chi shao)*, Cortex Moutan Radicis *(mu dan pi)*, and Radix et Caulis Jixueteng *(ji xue teng)* invigorate the blood and remove blood stasis. Radix Paeoniae Rubrae *(chi shao)* and Cortex Moutan Radicis *(mu dan pi)* also clear heat due to the yin deficiency. Periostracum Cicadae *(chan tui)* enters the Liver channel, where it expels wind and heat to relieve the itching.

MECHANISM OF ACTION: Herbs which act on the Kidneys, Liver, and Spleen are used to stimulate the immune and endocrine systems, whose failure in older women causes local dystrophy. The herbs prescribed for blood stasis serve to improve local blood flow and microcirculation; more oxygen and nutrients are thereby brought to the affected areas. This has the effect of helping normal tissue growth and preventing infections. The "white lesions" may even gradually subside if treatment is continued for six to twelve months.

EFFICACY: Over 90% of patients benefit from this approach. Better results can be obtained by combining the fumigation and sitz bath with the oral decoction. In one clinical study it was shown that the "white lesions" disappeared after three to six months of treatment in 30.5% of cases.

Acupuncture treatment

STRATEGY: Promote the smooth flow of qi and blood in the vulvar area, and regulate any imbalance among the Liver, Kidney, and Spleen channels.

MAIN POINTS: CV-1 *(hui yin)*, CV-3 *(zhong ji)*

ADDITIONAL POINTS: LR-3 *(tai chong)*, SP-6 *(san yin jiao)*, KI-3 *(tai xi)*, SP-10 *(xue hai)*

ANALYSIS OF PRESCRIPTION: The Conception vessel originates in the perineum and Womb. Points at the vulva and the lower abdomen are therefore especially responsive for diseases in that area, as they are local points that also belong to the involved channels. Neurovascular, neuroendocrine, and neuroimmune regulation mechanisms are involved in relieving the symptoms, including the "white lesions." Severe itching may result from Liver fire where the patient presents with a red tongue, thirst, irritability, and dark urine. In such cases, LR-3 *(tai chong)* with a reducing method is indicated in order to clear excessive heat from the Liver. In chronic cases, SP-10 *(xue hai)* is used to remove blood stasis. SP-6 *(san yin jiao)*,and KI-3 *(tai xi)* are used to tonify the yin when the tongue is red and the patient is thirsty.

EFFICACY: In one study, after three to six months patients showed an improvement in the lesions in 59% of cases, with little change in the others. Complete recovery occurred in 18.2% of cases.

Vulvar Pruritus

Pruritus is the most common symptom of vulvar disease. It consists of intense itching in the vulvar skin or mucosa, attributable to many causes. Specific diagnosis depends on a thorough history, a physical examination of the whole surface of the body, and, in most cases, adequate biopsy. Beside infection as an obvious cause, vulvar pruritus may be caused by local dystrophy, chemical substances such as contraceptive agents, wearing heat-retaining clothing, irritation from sweat, urine, or feces (often from fistulae), as well as systemic diseases such as diabetes, jaundice, nutritional deficiency, and psychiatric disorders. Prevention is thus largely a matter of patient education. Treatment is based on removing the causative factor. Keeping the area dry should be emphasized. Aside from specific therapy, symptomatic treatment such as antihistamines, mild sedatives, and topical lotions or powders can prove useful.

According to traditional Chinese medicine, vulvar pruritus can be differentiated into two categories. The first is heat excess in the Liver, which impairs the Spleen's ability to transform dampness. This results in dampness and heat pouring downward and accumulating in the vulvar area. The second diagnostic category is deficiency of the Liver and Kidneys. This causes the stirring of internal wind and heat, and insufficiency of blood and essence in the vulvar area.

Herbal treatment

Refer to Vulvar Dystrophy Formula 1 above. This formula is especially useful if the diagnosis is Liver fire or damp-heat pouring downward.

EFFICACY: Symptoms are generally relieved in one to two weeks. For better results, an additional two weeks of treatment are recommended.

Vulvar Pruritus Formula 1

This formula is indicated for chronic cases, and is taken orally. In severe cases, combine it with the fumigation and sitz bath method.

Radix Rehmanniae Glutinosae *(sheng di huang)* 12g

Fructus Corni Officinalis *(shan zhu yu)* 9g

Herba Epimedii *(yin yang huo)* 12g

Fructus Psoraleae Corylifoliae *(bu gu zhi)* 12g

Radix Clematidis *(wei ling xian)* 12g

Fructus Cnidii Monnieri *(she chuang zi)* 12g

Cortex Moutan Radicis *(mu dan pi)* 9g

Radix Paeoniae Rubrae *(chi shao)* 12g

Cooked Radix et Rhizoma Rhei *(zhi da huang)* 9g

ANALYSIS OF FORMULA: Radix Rehmanniae Glutinosae *(sheng di huang)*, Fructus Corni Officinalis *(shan zhu yu)*, Herba Epimedii *(yin yang huo)*, and Fructus Psoraleae Corylifoliae *(bu gu zhi)* nourish the Liver and Kidneys, thereby replenishing the essence and blood. Radix Clematidis *(wei ling xian)* is effective in removing wind and dampness from the channels. Fructus Cnidii Monnieri *(she chuang zi)* strengthens the Kidneys, dries dampness, and relieves itching. Cortex Moutan Radicis *(mu dan pi)*, Radix Paeoniae Rubrae *(chi shao)*, and Radix et Rhizoma Rhei *(da huang)* are used to expel heat and invigorate the blood, since blood stasis is often the cause of chronic vulvar pruritus.

MECHANISM OF ACTION: Radix Clematidis *(wei ling xian)* has analgesic and antibiotic properties. Fructus Cnidii Monnieri *(she chuang zi)* was found to have estrogenic actions and antibiotic properties in vitro. Radix Rehmanniae Glutinosae *(sheng di huang)*, Fructus Corni Officinalis *(shan zhu yu)*, Herba Epimedii *(yin yang huo)*, and Fructus Psoraleae Corylifoliae *(bu gu zhi)* are effective mainly through their endocrine and immune properties. Cortex Moutan Radicis *(mu dan pi)*, Radix Paeoniae Rubrae *(chi shao)*, and Radix et Rhizoma Rhei *(da huang)* are used not only for stimulating microcirculation, but also for relieving pain by increasing blood beta-endorphin levels.

EFFICACY: In one study, symptoms were relieved after one to two weeks of treatment in 80-90% of patients. Better results can be obtained by combining this formula with the fumigation and sitz bath method.

Acupuncture treatment

Treatment is the same as for vulvar dystrophy. If intense heat is present, TB-5 *(wai guan)* can be added to expel heat from the three Burners.

EFFICACY: In several clinical trials, 96.4% of patients have benefitted after two to three months treatment. Fifty percent were completely cured.

4

Inflammatory Diseases

Vulvitis

VULVITIS MAY BE caused by irritation attributable to a variety of factors including leukorrhea, urine, stools, sexually transmitted infection, specific or unspecific infections, diabetes mellitus, and even exposure to radiation. Symptoms are leukorrhea, intense itching, and dypareunia. Chronic vulvitis may cause such epithelial changes as thickening, chapping, or eczema. Treatment should be directed at removing the cause. Coitus should be avoided until cure has been achieved. Recurrent infections require treatment of the sexual partner. Concomitant vulvar pruritus may be treated conventionally with local application of a lotion or non-oily cream containing a corticosteroid, but chafing should be avoided.

Traditional Chinese medicine views the diagnosis and treatment of this condition identically to that of vulvar pruritus, discussed in the preceding chapter.

Bartholinitis and Bartholin's Cyst and Abscess

Gonococci or other bacteria may obstruct the Bartholin's duct, causing the retention of the gland's secretion and its dilatation. Secondary infection may then cause a recurrent abscess. Small, noninflamed cysts are asymptomatic. Symptoms of infection are pain, tenderness, and dyspareunia. Around the fluctuant mass, tissues become edematous and inflamed. In conventional medicine, primary treatment consists of appropriate antibiotic administration and marsupialization (a form of surgical drainage).

The traditional Chinese diagnosis is that of damp-heat pouring downward. In addition to systemic antibiotics, the juice of fresh, juicy, local Chinese herbs are applied. Herbs that eliminate heat and toxins are more effective fresh than in dried form. Commonly used herbs include:

Herba Cammelina Communis *(ya zhi cao)*
Herba Plantaginis *(che qian cao)*
Herba Taraxaci Mongolici cum Radice *(pu gong ying)*
Herba cum Radice Violae Yedoensitis *(zi hua di ding)*
Herba Portulacae Oleraceae *(ma chi xian)*

PREPARATION: Take a sufficient quantity of one or more of the fresh herbs and pound them into a paste. Apply locally and retain, changing the mixture three times per day until infection subsides. If fresh herbs are unavailable, it is possible to decoct dry herbs and apply them as a wash, or use them in a sitz bath. (This is a rural Chinese folk remedy, the efficacy of which has not been documented.)

Vaginitis

Vaginitis is typically caused by a variety of organisms: bacteria, viruses, *Candida albicans, Trichomonas,* and *Chlamydia trachomatis,* among others. This is often brought about by contamination, such as sexual transmission. When menopause or a systemic disorder is present, these organisms easily overwhelm the normal vaginal flora. Excessive vaginal discharge, pain, pruritus, and dyspareunia are the main symptoms.

In conventional medicine, treatment is directed at removing the causative factor; the sexual partner, if found positive, is treated as well. Specific antibiotics are used for specific types of organisms, and an estrogenic pessary is used for atrophic vaginitis.

Traditional Chinese medicine relies on the nature of the vaginal discharge as a diagnostic tool. A large amount of leukorrhea signifies deficiency of the Kidneys and Spleen. The color is interpreted as follows:

Yellow (especially if the discharge is smelly): damp-heat
Green: Liver constraint
Red (bloody): heat
Dark red ("black"): blood stasis

Deficiency of the Kidneys, Spleen, and Liver leads to the production of internal heat and dampness, which pours downward into the reproductive tract. Usually it is Kidney and Liver deficiency that generates heat, while deficiency of the Spleen leads to dampness. At present, herbal treatment applied either orally or as a douche produces good results in atrophic or recurrent vaginitis.

Vaginitis Formula 1: Local Application

Radix Arnebiae seu Lithospermi *(zi cao)* 15g
Cortex Phellodendri *(huang bai)* 12g
Radix Sophorae Flavescentis *(ku shen)* 12g
Alumen Praeparatum *(ku fan)* 9g
Fructus Cnidii Monnieri *(she chuang zi)* 15g
Fructus Kochiae Scopariae *(di fu zi)* 15g
Pericarpium Zanthoxyli Bungeani *(chuan jiao)* 9g

METHOD: Boil for fifteen minutes, expose the vulva to the fumes, and then use as a sitz bath twice a day for two weeks.

Vaginitis Formula 2: Complementary Treatment

Rhizoma Anemarrhenae Asphodeloidis *(zhi mu)* 12g
Cortex Phellodendri *(huang bai)* 12g
Radix Pseudostellariae Heterophyllae *(tai zi shen)* 15g
Radix Rehmanniae Glutinosae *(sheng di huang)* 15g

Carapax Amydae Sinensis *(bie jia)*..................................... 15g
Herba Epimedii *(yin yang huo)* 12g
Rhizoma Polygonati *(huang jing)*....................................... 12g
Fructus Cnidii Monnieri *(she chuang zi)* 12g
Rhizoma Dioscoreae Hypoglaucae *(bei xie)*............................. 12g

METHOD: Take daily as a decoction for two weeks.

ANALYSIS OF BOTH FORMULAS: Cortex Phellodendri *(huang bai)* eliminates heat and dampness, especially from the lower part of the body, and
relieves fire toxicity. Radix Arnebiae seu Lithospermi *(zi cao)* relieves fire
toxicity and cools the blood, and is useful for relieving vaginal itching.
Alumen Praeparatum *(ku fan)* relieves pathogenic inflammation and
swelling. Fructus Cnidii Monnieri *(she chuang zi)* tonifies the Kidneys,
expels cold and dampness from the vulva, and has useful antiparasitic
properties. Combined with herbs that clear heat, it expels damp-heat as
well. Fructus Kochiae Scopariae *(di fu zi)* and Radix Sophorae Flavescentis
(ku shen) are both antiparasitic and relieve itching. Pericarpium Zanthoxyli Bungeani *(chuan jiao)* dispels cold and kills parasites. All the herbs
used in the sitz bath show bacteriostatic activity.

In the decoction, Rhizoma Dioscoreae Hypoglaucae *(bei xie)* clears
heat from the lower part of the body and removes dampness through
diuresis. The other ingredients tonify the Kidneys, Spleen, and Liver and
are discussed elsewhere.

MECHANISM OF ACTION: The herbs used in the sitz bath have antibiotic,
antifugal, and antiparasitic actions in vitro. Most herbs in the decoction
play a role in relieving the itching or swelling, or in regulating the
endocrine and immune systems to help combat chronic infection.

EFFICACY: In one study, both formulas used in conjunction for two weeks
showed an efficacy rate of 80%.

Cervicitis

Acute and chronic cervicitis are the most common gynecologic diseases.
Acute cervicitis is often secondary to acute vaginitis, and is mainly trans-

mitted sexually. In chronic cervicitis, uterine cervical lacerations during delivery or eversion of the endocervical mucosa are nearly always the basis for indolent (slow-healing) inflammatory conditions. Lumbar pain and leukorrhea are the usual symptoms. In acute cases the discharge may be purulent, malodorous, and blood-tinged, and the patient may experience lower abdominal pain and dyspareunia, among other symptoms.

In conventional medicine the acute case is treated with local and systemic antibiotics. Chronic cases require a cervical smear, colposcopy, and biopsy in order to rule out cervical dysplasia or malignancy. Treatment usually consists of drug therapy, cauterization, laser or conventional surgery, or cryosugery.

Traditionally, Chinese medicine views acute cervicitis as damp-heat pouring downward. Chronic cervicitis is usually associated with deficiency of the Spleen.

Cervicitis Formula 1: Local Application

Rhizoma Pinelliae Ternatae Recens *(xian ban xia)* 1g

METHOD: Pound the fresh herb to express its juice, and soak the end of a vaginal tampon in the juice. Pack the tampon to the cervix for twenty-four hours, twice a week. Four weeks constitutes one course of treatment. Using the prepared dried herb gives no results. When the fresh herb is unavailable, substitute an extract of Rhizoma Pinelliae Ternatae Crudum *(sheng ban xia)*. NOTE: Both the fresh and untreated forms of this herb are extremely toxic. They should *never* be given orally, and instructions to patients in their use must be very clear.

ANALYSIS OF FORMULA: Rhizoma Pinelliae Ternatae Crudum *(sheng ban xia)* dispels dampness and resolves phlegm, which is useful in treating the inflammation caused by heat and dampness, and also in helping dissolve masses, which is the basis of cancer prevention.

MECHANISM OF ACTION: Rhizoma Pinelliae Ternatae Crudum *(sheng ban xia)* has a proven bacteriostatic effect on staphylococcus and colibacillus strains.

EFFICACY: In one study of 1349 patients, 75% obtained good results after several courses of the above treatment.

Cervicitis Formula 2: Complementary Treatment

STRATEGY: Strengthen the Spleen qi and tonify the Kidneys.

Radix Codonopsitis Pilosulae *(dang shen)* 12g
Radix Astragali Membranacei *(huang qi)* 12g
Rhizoma Atractylodis Macrocephalae *(bai zhu)* 9g
Rhizoma Atractylodis *(cang zhu)* 9g
Radix Dioscoreae Oppositae *(shan yao)* 12g
Sclerotium Poriae Cocos *(fu ling)* 12g
Herba Epimedii *(yin yang huo)* 12g
Rhizoma Polygonati *(huang jing)* 12g
Os Sepiae seu Sepiellae *(hai piao xiao)* 12g
Cortex Ailanthi Altissimae *(chun pi)* 12g

METHOD: Take daily as a decoction for four weeks.

ANALYSIS OF FORMULA: Radix Codonopsitis Pilosulae *(dang shen)*, Radix Astragali Membranacei *(huang qi)*, Rhizoma Atractylodis Macrocephalae *(bai zhu)*, and Radix Dioscoreae Oppositae *(shan yao)* are the principal herbs used to address the Spleen deficiency. One of the Spleen's transportive functions relates to the circulation of water, as it cannot tolerate dampness ("earth controls water"). Herba Epimedii *(yin yang huo)* and Rhizoma Polygonati *(huang jing)* tonify the Kidneys and strengthen the Spleen. Os Sepiae seu Sepiellae *(hai piao xiao)* and Cortex Ailanthi Altissimae *(chun pi)* check profuse leukorrhea.

MECHANISM OF ACTION: The herbs which strengthen the Spleen work by regulating the immune system. They also reduce blood viscosity, as shown by thromboxane B_2 levels.

Pelvic Inflammatory Disease (PID)

Introduction

High incidence and potentially serious consequences make PID the most important problem encoutered in gynecologic practice. Doctors are confronted with a wide variety of pelvic infections such as salpingo-oophoritis, tubo-ovarian abscess, pelvic abscess, pelvic cellulitis, and pelvic peritonitis. Endometritis usually occurs in the postpartum period in women with a history of PID. Recurrent pelvic infection adversely affects fertility. Ten percent of women affected with one episode of pelvic inflammation become infertile. The percentage increases to 25% after a second episode, and to 60% after a third episode. The pathogens are commonly polymicrobial with mixed aerobic and anaerobic bacteria. *Neisseria gonorhoeae* and *Chlamydia trachomatis* are frequent causative agents of salpingitis. An intrauterine device (IUD) is also a frequent cause of recurrent or chronic pelvic infection. Antibiotics are the treatment of choice in conventional medicine, especially in acute cases. Extirpative surgery or drainage is eventually necessary for pelvic abscess.

From a traditional perspective, PID may fall into one of several categories: heat penetrating the Womb, abdominal mass, leukorrhea, or menstrual pain. It usually results from dampness and heat toxin remaining in the Womb and in the Conception and Penetrating vessels, causing stagnancy of qi and blood. Later a mass may develop.

Depending upon the signs and symptoms, PID may be acute or chronic. In either form, it is always a complicated problem for patient and practitioner alike. Combination treatment using herbs and antibiotics together is much more effective than either treatment alone. As will be explained below, herbal treatment can take the form of a decoction, poultice, or enema. Combining different methods will yield better results. Herbal formulas should, of course, be modified when necessary to fit the patient's signs and symptoms.

Pelvic Inflammatory Disease: Acute

Acute Pelvic Inflammatory Disease Formula 1

INDICATIONS: High fever, chills, abdominal tenderness, nausea, vomiting, constipation or diarrhea, profuse yellowish and malodorous leukorrhea, dyspareunia, dark urine, thirst, dry tongue with a thick yellow coat, big and rapid pulse. In terms of the four-level differential diagnostic method, this pattern corresponds to pathogenic heat entering the nutritive level.

STRATEGY: Clear the heat toxin, invigorate the blood, and remove the abscess.

Flos Lonicerae Japonicae *(jin yin hua)* 12g
Fructus Forsythiae Suspensae *(lian qiao)* 12g
Flos Carthami Tinctorii *(hong hua)* 9g
Herba cum Radice Patriniae *(bai jiang cao)* 30g
Radix Paeoniae Rubrae *(chi shao)* 12g
Herba Taraxaci Mongolici cum Radice *(pu gong ying)* 30g
Gummi Olibanum *(ru xiang)* 3g
Myrrha *(mo yao)* 3g
Herba cum Radix Cynanchi Paniculati *(xu chang qing)* 15g
Cortex Moutan Radicis *(mu dan pi)* 9g
Semen Persicae *(tao ren)* 12g
Semen Coicis Lachryma-jobi *(yi yi ren)* 15g
Fructus Meliae Toosendan *(chuan lian zi)* 12g
Rhizoma Corydalis Yanhusuo *(yan hu suo)* 12g

METHOD: Take daily as a decoction for the duration of the acute episode. NOTE: This formula should be used only as an adjunct to systemic antibiotics.

MODIFICATIONS:

1. With yellowish, smelly leukorrhea, add:

Rhizoma Smilacis Glabrae *(tu fu ling)* 15g

Radix Sophorae Flavescentis *(ku shen)* 12g

2. With constipation, add:
Cooked Radix et Rhizoma Rhei *(zhi da huang)* 9g

3. With diarrhea, add:
Radix Pulsatillae Chinensis *(bai tou weng)* 12g
Cortex Phellodendri *(huang bai)* 12g
Cortex Fraxini *(qin pi)* 12g

4. With dark urine, add:
Tips of Radix Glycyrrhizae Uralensis *(gan cao shao)* 6g
Caulis Mutong *(mu tong)* 6g

ANALYSIS OF FORMULA: Flos Lonicerae Japonicae *(jin yin hua)* and Fructus Forsythiae Suspensae *(lian qiao)* have a strong effect in clearing heat toxin. Flos Carthami Tinctorii *(hong hua)*, Radix Paeoniae Rubrae *(chi shao)*, Cortex Moutan Radicis *(mu dan pi)*, and Semen Persicae *(tao ren)* invigorate the blood; the first two herbs also have cooling properties. Herba cum Radice Patriniae *(bai jiang cao)*, Herba Taraxaci Mongolici cum Radice *(pu gong ying)*, and Semen Coicis Lachryma-jobi *(yi yi ren)* clear heat and eliminate pus. Gummi Olibanum *(ru xiang)* and Myrrha *(mo yao)* remove blood stasis and alleviate pain. Fructus Meliae Toosendan *(chuan lian zi)* and Rhizoma Corydalis Yanhusuo *(yan hu suo)* facilitate the circulation of qi and remove blood stasis to further relieve the pain. Rhizoma Smilacis Glabrae *(tu fu ling)* and Radix Sophorae Flavescentis *(ku shen)* remove dampness and heat from the lower part of the body. Cooked Radix et Rhizoma Rhei *(zhi da huang)* relieves constipation, expels internal heat, and removes blood stasis. Radix Pulsatillae Chinensis *(bai tou weng)*, Cortex Phellodendri *(huang bai)*, and Cortex Fraxini *(qin pi)* together relieve diarrhea and clear heat and dampness. Radix Glycyrrhizae Uralensis *(gan cao)* clears heat. Tips of Radix Glycyrrhizae Uralensis *(gan cao shao)*, together with Caulis Mutong *(mu tong)*, are used to clear heat through diuresis, which is indicated in urethritis.

MECHANISM OF ACTION: This formula acts in four different ways. First, it has broad-spectrum bacteriostatic activity for both aerobic and anaerobic organisms. Second, it improves microcirculation by regulating the flow of blood. Third, it has diuretic and purgative properties, which helps rid the body of toxins. And fourth, it also strengthens the immune system to help fight the infection.

EFFICACY: This formula, in combination with antibiotics, is much more effective than antibiotics alone.

Acute Pelvic Inflammatory Disease Formula 2

INDICATIONS: Dampness and heat pouring downward, as indicated by lower abdominal tenderness, fluctuating low fever, profuse yellowish leukorrhea, lumbosacral pain and soreness, red tongue with a yellow coating, and a rapid pulse. In terms of the four-level differential diagnostic method, this pattern corresponds to pathogenic heat entering the qi level.

Radix Scutellariae Baicalensis *(huang qin)* 12g
Cortex Phellodendri *(huang bai)* 12g
Rhizoma Coptidis *(huang lian)* 6g
Sclerotium Poriae Cocos *(fu ling)* 12g
Radix Glycyrrhizae Uralensis *(gan cao)* 6g
Rhizoma Alismatis Orientalis *(ze xie)* 9g
Herba cum Radice Patriniae *(bai jiang cao)* 15g
Fructus Meliae Toosendan *(chuan lian zi)* 12g
Rhizoma Corydalis Yanhusuo *(yan hu suo)* 15g
Cooked Radix et Rhizoma Rhei *(zhi da huang)* 9g
Herba cum Radix Cynanchi Paniculati *(xu chang qing)* 15g

METHOD: Take daily as a decoction for the duration of the acute episode.

MODIFICATIONS:

1. With unabating fever, add:
    Herba Artemisiae Yinchenhao *(yin chen hao)* 15g
    Fructus Gardeniae Jasminoidis *(zhi zi)* 12g
    Cortex Magnoliae Officinalis *(hou po)* 6g

2. With lumbar and sacral soreness, add:

Radix Achyranthis Bidentatae *(niu xi)* 9g

Radix Salviae Miltiorrhizae *(dan shen)* 12g

Radix Paeoniae Rubrae *(chi shao)* 12g

Cortex Moutan Radicis *(mu dan pi)* 9g

ANALYSIS OF FORMULA: Radix Scutellariae Baicalensis *(huang qin)*, Rhizoma Coptidis *(huang lian)*, and Cortex Phellodendri *(huang bai)* expel heat and dampness. Together they consitute the classical formula Three-Yellow Decoction *(san huang tang)*. Herba cum Radice Patriniae *(bai jiang cao)* clears heat and expels pus. Sclerotium Poriae Cocos *(fu ling)* and Rhizoma Alismatis Orientalis *(ze xie)* eliminate dampness through the urine. Fructus Meliae Toosendan *(chuan lian zi)*, Rhizoma Corydalis Yanhusuo *(yan hu suo)*, and Herba cum Radix Cynanchi Paniculati *(xu chang qing)* facilitate the flow of qi and remove blood stasis to eliminate the pain. Cooked Radix et Rhizoma Rhei *(zhi da huang)* clears heat and invigorates the blood. Radix Glycyrrhizae Uralensis *(gan cao)* is used here to mitigate the properties of the other herbs; it also helps relieve toxicity. Herba Artemisiae Yinchenhao *(yin chen hao)*, Fructus Gardeniae Jasminoidis *(zhi zi)*, and Cortex Magnoliae Officinalis *(hou po)* together drain damp-heat. Radix Achyranthis Bidentatae *(niu xi)*, Radix Salviae Miltiorrhizae *(dan shen)*, Radix Paeoniae Rubrae *(chi shao)*, and Cortex Moutan Radicis *(mu dan pi)* drain damp-heat that has accumulated in the channels of the back by invigorating the blood.

MECHANISM OF ACTION: This formula focuses on controlling organisms that are not as virulent as those addressed by the first formula, but that are more threatening to fertility. These are mostly gram-negative bacilli similar to those found in the normal intestinal flora. The diuretic and purgative properties of the decoction are similar to those in the first formula.

EFFICACY: This formula, in combination with antibiotics, is much more effective than antibiotics alone.

Pelvic Inflammatory Disease: Chronic

This condition is usually secondary to changes induced by a previous episode of acute PID. It may also present as an acute reinfection.

Chronic Pelvic Inflammatory Disease Formula 1

INDICATIONS: Signs and symptoms include lower abdominal pain or distention, lumbar or sacral soreness that is exacerbated around the time of menstruation or after intercourse, prolonged menstrual bleeding (up to 15 days), yellowish leukorrhea, a greasy yellow tongue coating, and a slippery pulse.

STRATEGY: Expel damp-heat, invigorate the blood, and clear the channels.

Radix Gentianae Longdancao *(long dan cao)* 15g
Herba Lycopi Lucidi *(ze lan)* 9g
Rhizoma Alismatis Orientalis *(ze xie)* 9g
Sclerotium Poriae Cocos *(fu ling)* 12g
Semen Persicae *(tao ren)* 12g
Semen Coicis Lachryma-jobi *(yi yi ren)* 15g
Fructus Gardeniae Jasminoidis *(zhi zi)* 12g
Cortex Moutan Radicis *(mu dan pi)* 9g
Radix Salviae Miltiorrhizae *(dan shen)* 12g
Radix Ligustici Chuanxiong *(chuan xiong)* 9g
Fructus Meliae Toosendan *(chuan lian zi)* 12g
Rhizoma Corydalis Yanhusuo *(yan hu suo)* 15g
Herba cum Radix Cynanchi Paniculati *(xu chang qing)* 15g

METHOD: Take daily as a decoction for three to six months.

MODIFICATIONS:

1. With obstructed fallopian tubes, add:
   Rhizoma Acori Graminei *(shi chang pu)* 15g

Fructus Liquidambaris Taiwanianae *(lu lu tong)* 12g
Semen Vaccariae Segetalis *(wang bu liu xing)* 12g
Lumbricus *(di long)*... 12g

2. With hydrosalpinx (fluid in the fallopian tubes), add:
Radix Astragali Membranacei *(huang qi)*............................. 12g
Radix Aristolochiae Fangchi *(fang ji)* 9g
Radix Achyranthis Bidentatae *(niu xi)*.............................. 12g
Semen Plantaginis *(che qian zi)*.................................... 12g

ANALYSIS OF FORMULA: Rhizoma Alismatis Orientalis *(ze xie)*, Sclerotium Poriae Cocos *(fu ling)*, and Semen Coicis Lachryma-jobi *(yi yi ren)* are used to remove the dampness. Herba Lycopi Lucidi *(ze lan)*, Semen Persicae *(tao ren)*, Radix Salviae Miltiorrhizae *(dan shen)*, Radix Ligustici Chuanxiong *(chuan xiong)*, and Cortex Moutan Radicis *(mu dan pi)* invigorate the blood as part of the same strategy of removing dampness. Cortex Moutan Radicis *(mu dan pi)* also clears the heat, along with Radix Gentianae Longdancao *(long dan cao)* and Fructus Gardeniae Jasminoidis *(zhi zi)*. Fructus Meliae Toosendan *(chuan lian zi)*, Rhizoma Corydalis Yanhusuo *(yan hu suo)*, and Herba cum Radix Cynanchi Paniculati *(xu chang qing)* promote the flow of qi to relieve the pain, and further contribute to eliminating the dampness. Fructus Liquidambaris Taiwanianae *(lu lu tong)*, Semen Vaccariae Segetalis *(wang bu liu xing)*, Lumbricus *(di long)*, and Rhizoma Acori Graminei *(shi chang pu)* remove stubborn phlegm and dissolve masses. Radix Astragali Membranacei *(huang qi)*, Radix Aristolochiae Fangchi *(fang ji)*, Radix Achyranthis Bidentatae *(niu xi)*, and Semen Plantaginis *(che qian zi)* are strong water expellants. The function of Radix Astragali Membranacei *(huang qi)* is noteworthy: its strengthening of the qi significantly helps the other herbs move water.

MECHANISM OF ACTION: Chronic infection usually shows a predominance of dampness and blood stasis. The herbs in this formula are not bacteriostatic, but are aimed at changing the internal environment so that it is no longer favorable to infection. This may help improve the patient's microcirculation, organic functions, and immune system. Appetite and sleep may improve as well. The result would be to enable the body to fight the pathogenic organisms more effectively with the help of antibiotics.

EFFICACY: Most patients will recover sooner if they take this formula in combination with antibiotics than if they take antibiotics alone. If the fallopian tubes are completely blocked, especially as a sequela of tuberculosis, there is little hope of recovering tubal patency. When the tubes are blocked proximally and of recent date, some patients may get results. Best results are obtained when blockage is incomplete (as demonstrated by hysterosalpingography) and due to infection or adhesion.

Chronic Pelvic Inflammatory Disease Formula 2

INDICATIONS: Blood stasis with cold, showing as abdominal pain relieved by warmth, lumbosacral soreness, a sensation of heaviness or being weighed down, aggravation of symptoms during menstruation, scanty menstruation, a bluish tongue with spots and a thin coating, and a fine pulse.

STRATEGY: Invigorate the blood using herbs with warm properties.

Radix Bupleuri *(chai hu)* 9g
Radix Angelicae Sinensis *(dang gui)* 12g
Radix Ligustici Chuanxiong *(chuan xiong)* 12g
Fructus Foeniculi Vulgaris *(xiao hui xiang)* 12g
Cortex Cinnamomi Cassiae *(rou gui)* 3g
Squama Manitis Pentadactylae *(chuan shan jia)* 12g
Radix Salviae Miltiorrhizae *(dan shen)* 12g
Radix Achyranthis Bidentatae *(niu xi)* 12g
Rhizoma Corydalis Yanhusuo *(yan hu suo)* 12g
Pollen Typhae *(pu huang)* 12g
Excrementum Trogopterori seu Pteromi *(wu ling zhi)* 12g
Radix Linderae Strychnifoliae *(wu yao)* 9g

METHOD: Take daily as a decoction for three to six months.

MODIFICATIONS:

1. With scanty menses, add:
   Radix et Caulis Jixueteng *(ji xue teng)* 15g
   Herba Leonuri Heterophylli *(yi mu cao)* 12g
   Herba Lycopi Lucidi *(ze lan)* 12g

2. With an infectious mass, add:
   Rhizoma Sparganii Stoloniferi *(san leng)* 12g
   Rhizoma Curcumae Ezhu *(e zhu)* 12g
   Spina Gleditsiae Sinensis *(zao jiao ci)* 12g
   Radix Rubiae Cordifoliae *(qian cao gen)* 12g

ANALYSIS OF FORMULA: Radix Angelicae Sinensis *(dang gui)*, Radix Ligustici Chuanxiong *(chuan xiong)*, and Radix Salviae Miltiorrhizae *(dan shen)* invigorate the blood. Radix Achyranthis Bidentatae *(niu xi)*, Pollen Typhae *(pu huang)*, and Excrementum Trogopteri seu Pteromi *(wu ling zhi)* dispel blood stasis. Squama Manitis Pentadactylae *(chuan shan jia)* dissolves masses and resolves phlegm. Radix Bupleuri *(chai hu)*, Fructus Foeniculi Vulgaris *(xiao hui xiang)*, and Radix Linderae Strychnifoliae *(wu yao)* promote the flow of qi; Radix Bupleuri *(chai hu)* is cool, while the other two have warm properties. Cortex Cinnamomi Cassiae *(rou gui)* expels cold and relieves pain better than Ramulus Cinnamomi Cassiae *(gui zhi)*. Radix et Caulis Jixueteng *(ji xue teng)* and Herba Lycopi Lucidi *(ze lan)* remove blood stasis from the channels. Herba Leonuri Heterophylli *(yi mu cao)* removes blood stasis from the Womb. Rhizoma Sparganii Stoloniferi *(san leng)*, Rhizoma Curcumae Ezhu *(e zhu)*, and Spina Gleditsiae Sinensis *(zao jiao ci)* dissolve masses, while Radix Rubiae Cordifoliae *(qian cao gen)* invigorates the blood and eliminates stasis.

MECHANISM OF ACTION: This formula regulates the microcirculation, improves tissue edema, and helps fight infection. It also helps improve circulation by relieving pain and muscle spasms.

EFFICACY: In combination with antibiotics, this is an important formula for treating PID. Some studies have demonstrated that 70-80% of patients thus treated have shown significant improvement.

Chronic Pelvic Inflammatory Disease Formula 3

INDICATIONS: Stagnancy of qi and blood, as shown by lower abdominal pain or distention, irritability, breast tenderness before menses, leukorrhea, constipation, wiry pulse, and a dark tongue with little coating.

STRATEGY: Promote the flow of qi and invigorate the blood in order to free the channels.

Cortex Moutan Radicis *(mu dan pi)* 9g
Radix Salviae Miltiorrhizae *(dan shen)* 15g
Radix Paeoniae Rubrae *(chi shao)* 12g
Radix Ligustici Chuanxiong *(chuan xiong)* 9g
Rhizoma Cyperi Rotundi *(xiang fu)* 12g
Radix Rubiae Cordifoliae *(qian cao gen)* 12g
Semen Persicae *(tao ren)* 12g
Rhizoma Corydalis Yanhusuo *(yan hu suo)* 12g
Fructus Meliae Toosendan *(chuan lian zi)* 12g
Semen Citri Reticulatae *(ju he)* 6g
Treated Carapax Amydae Sinensis *(zhi bie jia)* 12g

METHOD: Take daily as a decoction for three to six months.

MODIFICATION: With premenstrual breast engorgement, add:
Fructus Liquidambaris Taiwanianae *(lu lu tong)* 12g
Tuber Curcumae *(yu jin)* 12g

ANALYSIS OF FORMULA: Radix Salviae Miltiorrhizae *(dan shen)*, Radix Paeoniae Rubrae *(chi shao)*, Radix Ligustici Chuanxiong *(chuan xiong)*, Radix Rubiae Cordifoliae *(qian cao gen)*, and Semen Persicae *(tao ren)* invigorate the blood and dispel blood stasis. Cortex Moutan Radicis *(mu dan pi)* both cools and invigorates the blood. Rhizoma Cyperi Rotundi *(xiang fu)* and Rhizoma Corydalis Yanhusuo *(yan hu suo)* promote the flow of qi in the reproductive tract. Semen Citri Reticulatae *(ju he)* and treated Carapax Amydae Sinensis *(zhi bie jia)* remove stagnant qi and phlegm from the Liver channel. The latter ingredient is baked with a little vinegar to strengthen its ability to remove phelgm and reduce masses. Fructus Liquidambaris Taiwanianae *(lu lu tong)* and Tuber Curcumae *(yu jin)* facilitate the flow of qi in the Liver channel, especially in the breasts.

MECHANISM OF ACTION: This formula not only relieves pelvic pain and calms the patient, but also softens chronically infected tissues. For example, Semen Persicae *(tao ren)* has proven fibrolytic action in vitro.

EFFICACY: With the appropriate presentation, patients treated with this formula in combination with antibiotics can expect relief in 80% of cases.

Chronic Pelvic Inflammatory Disease Formula 4: Poultice

STRATEGY: Locally clear the heat, invigorate the blood, and remove the dampness.

Radix et Rhizoma Notopterygii *(qiang huo)* 15g
Radix Angelicae Pubescentis *(du huo)*................................15g
Radix Angelicae Dahuricae *(bai zhi)*................................12g
Radix Ledebouriellae Divaricatae *(fang feng)* 18g
Radix Lateralis Aconiti Carmichaeli Praeparata *(fu zi)*..................9g
Radix Gentianae Qinjiao *(qin jiao)* 21g
Herba cum Radice Lycopodii Clavati *(shen jin cao)* 30g
Herba Speranskiae seu Impatientis *(tou gu cao)* 30g
Radix et Caulis Jixueteng *(ji xue teng)*................................30g
Folium Artemisiae Argyi *(ai ye)* 30g

METHOD: Grind to a coarse powder, place in a muslin bag, and steam for 20 minutes. Apply on the lower abdomen for 30 minutes or until the bag has cooled down. Administer once daily, except when menstruating, for three to six months. The same bag can be used for six or seven days.

ANALYSIS OF FORMULA: These herbs are aromatic and transform dampness. They are warm, invigorate the flow of qi and blood in the channels, and remove phlegm.

MECHANISM OF ACTION: The recovery of infectious tissues is helped by relieving venous congestion in the pelvic area through the invigoration of the qi and blood.

EFFICACY: Patients with chronic PID experience great symptomatic relief, especially from pain and leukorrhea.

Chronic Pelvic Inflammatory Disease Formula 5: Enema

STRATEGY: Clear the heat from the pelvic cavity and invigorate the blood through a kind of peritoneodialysis by way of the colon.

Flos Carthami Tinctorii *(hong hua)* 30g
Herba cum Radice Patriniae *(bai jiang cao)* 30g
Herba Taraxaci Mongolici cum Radice *(pu gong ying)* 15g
Herba cum Radice Violae Yedoensitis *(zi hua di ding)* 15g
Radix Salviae Miltiorrhizae *(dan shen)* 12g
Radix Paeoniae Rubrae *(chi shao)* 12g

METHOD: Make a 100ml concentrated decoction. Bring the concentrate to about 98-104°F (37-40°C). The enema tube should enter 8 inches (20cm) into the rectum. Slowly drip the entire decoction into the rectum over five to six minutes. Administer every evening except when menstruating. Better results will be obtained if the medicine is not rapidly expelled. It is possible to prepare the decoction for three to four days in advance if it is kept refrigerated.

ANALYSIS OF FORMULA: All of the herbs invigorate the blood and/or have bacteriostatic actions in vitro.

MECHANISM OF ACTION: Applied in this method, the herbs will permeate the pelvic blood stream directly and at a high concentration.

EFFICACY: Roughly the same as for the poultice described above.

Gonorrhea

The columnar and transitional epithelia of the genitourinary tract are the principal sites of invasion for *Neisseria gonorrhoae*. This organism may enter the upper reproductive tract, causing salpingitis and its attendant complications. About 80% of women with gonorrhea are asymptomatic. Even when symptoms occur, they are much milder than in the male. Early symptoms are localized in the lower genitourinary tract, and include purulent vaginal discharge, urinary frequency or dysuria, and rectal discomfort. The vulvar area may itch or burn. Bartholinitis is sometimes a complication. A presumptive diagnosis can be made based on microscopic examination of the stained smear. Large doses of penicilin are the conventional treatment of choice.

In traditional Chinese medicine, gonorrhea falls in the general category of urinary disturbance with turbid discharge. Depending on the symptoms, it is generally regarded as dampness and heat in the Lower Burner. Besides local complaints, patients present with fever, dark urine, a red tongue, and a rapid pulse. Herbal treatment in addition to antibiotics may be the best therapy. When the acute symptoms have subsided, patients may complain of lumbar pain and similar symptoms, which reflect the chronic stage of the disorder with residual heat and yin deficiency.

Gonorrhea Formula 1

STRATEGY: Eliminate toxic heat and dampness (acute illness).

Rhizoma Smilacis Glabrae *(tu fu ling)* 30g
Semen Coicis Lachryma-jobi *(yi yi ren)* 30g
Herba Artemisiae Yinchenhao *(yin chen hao)* 30g
Rhizoma Imperatae Cylindricae *(bai mao gen)* 30g
Talcum *(hua shi)* 20g
Tips of Radix Glycyrrhizae Uralensis *(gan cao shao)* 10g
Radix Scutellariae Baicalensis *(huang qin)* 10g
Cortex Phellodendri *(huang bai)* 15g

Rhizoma Coptidis *(huang lian)* 10g
Fructus Gardeniae Jasminoidis *(zhi zi)* 15g
Flos Lonicerae Japonicae *(jin yin hua)* 20g
Fructus Forsythiae Suspensae *(lian qiao)* 20g

MODIFICATIONS:

1. With constipation, add:
   Cooked Radix et Rhizoma Rhei *(zhi da huang)* 10g

2. With intense heat, add:
   Gypsum *(shi gao)* 10g
   Rhizoma Anemarrhenae Asphodeloidis *(zhi mu)* 15g

3. With heat and dampness, add:
   Semen Plantaginis *(che qian zi)* 15g
   Radix Gentianae Longdancao *(long dan cao)* 10g

ANALYSIS OF FORMULA: Rhizoma Smilacis Glabrae *(tu fu ling)* eliminates toxic heat and dampness. According to the traditional literature, this herb has been used for sexually transmitted diseases such as syphilis. Semen Coicis Lachryma-jobi *(yi yi ren)* and Talcum *(hua shi)* clear damp-heat through diuresis. Herba Artemisiae Yinchenhao *(yin chen hao)*, Radix Gentianae Longdancao *(long dan cao)*, Rhizoma Imperatae Cylindricae *(bai mao gen)*, and Herba Plantaginis *(che qian cao)* are effective in removing heat and dampness. Radix Scutellariae Baicalensis *(huang qin)*, Cortex Phellodendri *(huang bai)*, and Rhizoma Coptidis *(huang lian)* expel heat, especially from each of the three Burners. Flos Lonicerae Japonicae *(jin yin hua)*, Fructus Gardeniae Jasminoidis *(zhi zi)*, and Fructus Forsythiae Suspensae *(lian qiao)* clear toxic heat and cool the blood. Radix Glycyrrhizae Uralensis *(gan cao)* harmonizes the formula and clears toxic heat. The tips are popular for treating urinary disorders. In some cases interior heat may cause constipation, which leads to food stagnation. Internal heat also consumes the qi, which can lead to blood stasis. Cooked Radix et Rhizoma Rhei *(zhi da huang)* is therefore added as a purgative and antidote to eliminate the toxic heat, and resolve the stagnant food and blood stasis. Rhizoma Anemarrhenae Asphodeloidis *(zhi mu)* helps Gypsum *(shi gao)* clear the heat, especially when it is accompanied by yin deficiency with great thirst.

MECHANISM OF ACTION: The mechanism of action in this formula has yet to be explained. In general, these herbs are anti-inflammatory in three ways. First, they suppress the growth of bacteria. Herbs in this group include Rhizoma Smilacis Glabrae *(tu fu ling)*, Herba Artemisiae Yinchenhao *(yin chen hao)*, Flos Lonicerae Japonicae *(jin yin hua)*, Fructus Forsythiae Suspensae *(lian qiao)*, Radix Scutellariae Baicalensis *(huang qin)*, Rhizoma Coptidis *(huang lian)*, Cortex Phellodendri *(huang bai)*, and Rhizoma Imperatae Cylindricae *(bai mao gen)*. Second, they regulate the immune system. Herbs such as Herba Artemisiae Yinchenhao *(yin chen hao)*, Radix Glycyrrhizae Uralensis *(gan cao)*, Radix Scutellariae Baicalensis *(huang qin)*, and Radix et Rhizoma Rhei *(da huang)* share this function. Third, they improve the circulation of blood. In this group we find Radix et Rhizoma Rhei *(da huang)*, Fructus Gardeniae Jasminoidis *(zhi zi)*, Radix Scutellariae Baicalensis *(huang qin)*, and Rhizoma Coptidis *(huang lian)*.

Gonorrhea Formula 2

STRATEGY: Nourish the Kidneys and eliminate residual toxic heat (chronic illness).

Radix Rehmanniae Glutinosae Conquitae *(shu di huang)* 20g
Fructus Corni Officinalis *(shan zhu yu)* 15g
Radix Dioscoreae Oppositae *(shan yao)* 30g
Rhizoma Dioscoreae Hypoglaucae *(bei xie)* 12g
Semen Plantaginis *(che qian zi)* 12g
Rhizoma Smilacis Glabrae *(tu fu ling)* 15g
Semen Coicis Lachryma-jobi *(yi yi ren)* 15g
Rhizoma Alismatis Orientalis *(ze xie)* 15g
Radix Dipsaci Asperi *(xu duan)* 12g
Fructus Lycii *(gou qi zi)* 12g

Cortex Eucommiae Ulmoidis *(du zhong)*............................12g
Ootheca Mantidis *(sang piao xiao)*.........................9g

METHOD: Take daily as a decoction.

ANALYSIS OF FORMULA: Radix Rehmanniae Glutinosae Conquitae *(shu di huang)*, Fructus Corni Officinalis *(shan zhu yu)*, and Radix Dioscoreae Oppositae *(shan yao)* nourish the yin and the Kidneys. During the acute stage, toxic heat consumes the yin. In the later stage the body's resistance has been compromised, and residual toxic heat cannot be eliminated by heat-clearing herbs alone. Thus the approach here is to replenish the yin and the Kidneys, which really amounts to strengthening the endocrine and immune systems. Radix Dipsaci Asperi *(xu duan)*, Fructus Lycii *(gou qi zi)*, Cortex Eucommiae Ulmoidis *(du zhong)*, and Ootheca Mantidis *(sang piao xiao)* are special herbs for lumbar pain due to chronic illness and Kidney deficiency. Rhizoma Dioscoreae Hypoglaucae *(bei xie)*, Semen Plantaginis *(che qian zi)*, Rhizoma Smilacis Glabrae *(tu fu ling)*, Semen Coicis Lachryma-jobi *(yi yi ren)*, and Rhizoma Alismatis Orientalis *(ze xie)* are used mainly to eliminate heat and dampness.

MECHANISM OF ACTION: The mechanism of action in this formula has yet to be explained.

EFFICACY: When herbs are taken in addition to antibiotics, patients recover more quickly and more durably than when either herbs or antibiotics are used alone. Herbs are typically given for seven days in these cases. In one study using a seven-day treament involving almost 2000 patients (men and women) with gonorrhea, about two-thirds recovered with herbal treatment alone, while slightly over three-quarters recovered with a combination of antibiotics and herbal treatment. Recovery was defined as three consecutive weekly negative smears.

Endnote

1. Li Cunfu, "A review of herbal treatment for gonorrhea," *Research in Traditional Chinese Medicine*, 1994, 6:58-60.

5

Anovulatory Menstrual Disorders

MENSTRUAL DISORDERS DIFFER from the normal menstrual cycle in frequency, amount, or duration of flow. The term "menstrual disorder" is warranted when there are no organic changes. These disorders are divided into two categories: anovulatory and non-anovulatory. In this chapter we are concerned with anovulatory menstrual disorders.

Dysfunctional Uterine Bleeding

Dysfunctional uterine bleeding occurs mostly during puberty and the climacteric. Irregular bleeding with monophasic basal body temperature (BBT), proliferative endometrium, or endometrial hyperplasia may lead to anemia. Systemic diseases should be ruled out, and in premenopausal cases, endometrial carcinoma should be ruled out as well.

The treatment principle in conventional medicine is to stop the flow of blood, regularize the menstrual cycle, and, in young patients, to induce ovulation with hormone or hormone-like therapy.

In traditional Chinese medicine, reproduction is mainly dependent upon the Kidneys and its by-product, "heavenly dew" *(tian gui)*.

Originally, heavenly dew meant the water of the Kidneys, that is, their sexual regulatory function. A modern biomedical interpretation of heavenly dew is the positive and negative feedback loops of the hormonal sexual axis, whose function is established by the time a girl turns fourteen and her follicles are fully developed. Anovulatory dysfunctional uterine bleeding is caused primarily by deficiency of the Kidneys, and sometimes by Liver or Spleen deficiency as well. Puberty and the climacteric are periods when the Kidneys are immature or weakened. Blood loss in turn depletes the yin with resulting internal heat. Qi deficiency and blood stasis follow thereafter.

Herbal treatment

Hormones such as progestin are more effective and faster acting than herbs in stopping uterine bleeding. However, herbs are more effective in improving ovarian and pituitary function, alone or in combination with hormone therapy.

Dysfunctional Uterine Bleeding Formula 1

Radix Rehmanniae Glutinosae Conquitae *(shu di huang)* 12g
Radix Dioscoreae Oppositae *(shan yao)* 12g
Rhizoma Polygonati *(huang jing)* 9g
Herba Epimedii *(yin yang huo)* 12g
Radix Morindae Officinalis *(ba ji tian)* 12g
Fructus Corni Officinalis *(shan zhu yu)* 9g
Fructus Psoraleae Corylifoliae *(bu gu zhi)* 12g

METHOD: Take daily for three to six months.

MODIFICATIONS:

1. With internal heat, add:
   Rhizoma Anemarrhenae Asphodeloidis *(zhi mu)* 12g

Cortex Phellodendri *(huang bai)* 12g

Radix Scutellariae Baicalensis *(huang qin)* 12g

2. With qi deficiency, add:
Radix Codonopsitis Pilosulae *(dang shen)* 12g
Rhizoma Atractylodis Macrocephalae *(bai zhu)* 9g
Quick-fried Rhizoma Zingiberis Officinalis *(pao jiang)* 3g

3. With yang deficiency, add:
Radix Lateralis Aconiti Carmichaeli Praeparata *(fu zi)* 9g
Cortex Cinnamomi Cassiae *(rou gui)* 3g
Gelatinum Cornu Cervi *(lu jiao jiao)* 3g

ANALYSIS OF FORMULA: Radix Rehmanniae Glutinosae Conquitae *(shu di huang)*, Herba Epimedii *(yin yang huo)*, Radix Morindae Officinalis *(ba ji tian)*, Fructus Corni Officinalis *(shan zhu yu)*, Fructus Psoraleae Corylifoliae *(bu gu zhi)*, Radix Dioscoreae Oppositae *(shan yao)*, and Rhizoma Polygonati *(huang jing)* together are very effective in replenishing the Kidney yin and yang, especially the yang. They are warm in nature without being hot, tonify the Kidney essence, bring the sexual essence to maturity, and bring about the arrival of "heavenly dew" *(tian gui)*. The modifications are based on traditional differential diagnosis. Rhizoma Anemarrhenae Asphodeloidis *(zhi mu)*, Cortex Phellodendri *(huang bai)*, and Radix Scutellariae Baicalensis *(huang qin)* are used to reduce the internal heat, which results from the injury to the yin. Radix Codonopsitis Pilosulae *(dang shen)*, Rhizoma Atractylodis Macrocephalae *(bai zhu)*, and Quick-fried Rhizoma Zingiberis Officinalis *(pao jiang)* tonify the qi in order to generate more blood. Radix Lateralis Aconiti Carmichaeli Praeparata *(fu zi)*, Cortex Cinnamomi Cassiae *(rou gui)*, and Gelatinum Cornu Cervi *(lu jiao jiao)* should be used when the patient shows a loss of energy with intolerance of cold.

MECHANISM OF ACTION: This formula is most appropriate for patients showing normal FSH levels, but low estrogen levels and no ovulation. After treatment the patient's estrogen level rises, and BBT becomes biphasic again.

EFFICACY: In one study, for 73 out of 100 patients treated with herbs alone for three to six months, menstruation returned to normal with biphasic BBT.

Dysfunctional Uterine Bleeding Formula 2

Radix Codonopsitis Pilosulae *(dang shen)* 12g

Rhizoma Atractylodis Macrocephalae *(bai zhu)* 9g

Radix Rehmanniae Glutinosae Conquitae *(shu di huang)* 12g

Gelatinum Corii Asini *(e jiao)* 9g

Radix Paeoniae Lactiflorae *(bai shao)* 12g

Herba Agrimoniae Pilosae *(xian he cao)* 15g

Herba Epimedii *(yin yang huo)* 12g

Cacumen Biotae Orientalis *(ce bai ye)* 12g

Radix Sanguisorbae Officinalis *(di yu)* 12g

Radix Rubiae Cordifoliae *(qian cao gen)* 12g

Os Sepiae seu Sepiellae *(hai piao xiao)* 12g

Fructus Sophorae Japonicae Immaturus *(huai hua mi)* 12g

METHOD: Take as a decoction daily for two to three months.

ANALYSIS OF FORMULA: This formula is especially suited for dysfunctional uterine bleeding during the climacteric. Radix Codonopsitis Pilosulae *(dang shen)*, Rhizoma Atractylodis Macrocephalae *(bai zhu)*, Radix Rehmanniae Glutinosae Conquitae *(shu di huang)*, Gelatinum Corii Asini *(e jiao)*, Radix Paeoniae Lactiflorae *(bai shao)*, and Herba Agrimoniae Pilosae *(xian he cao)* are effective in replenishing the qi and blood in order to strengthen the uterine contractions. This helps control the bleeding. Herba Epimedii *(yin yang huo)*, Radix Rehmanniae Glutinosae Conquitae *(shu di huang)*, Gelatinum Corii Asini *(e jiao)*, and Radix Paeoniae Lactiflorae *(bai shao)* are used to tonify the Kidneys. Cacumen Biotae Orientalis *(ce bai ye)*, Radix Sanguisorbae Officinalis *(di yu)*, and Fructus Sophorae Japonicae Immaturus *(huai hua mi)* cool the blood and stop the bleeding. Radix Rubiae Cordifoliae *(qian cao gen)* invigorates the blood, while Os Sepiae seu Sepiellae *(hai piao xiao)* is used as an astringent. These two substances work synergistically to check the bleeding.

MECHANISM OF ACTION: Climacteric patients who experience dysfunctional uterine bleeding generally present with deficiency of the Kidneys, qi, and blood, complicated by blood stasis. In addition to anovulation, patients also exhibit endometrial changes. Endocrine imbalances may also indirectly affect endometrial prostaglandin levels, another factor in bleeding. Traditional treatment is beneficial not only for the ovaries, but also for the endometrium.

EFFICACY: Most patients will display regular bleeding cycles after traditional treatment alone. Sometimes it will be necessary to combine herbal treatment with progestin therapy, particularly in cases with endometrial hyperplasia.

Acupuncture treatment

In young patients it is appropriate to induce ovulation. The reader is referred to the section on inducing ovulation with acupuncture at the end of this chapter.

Polycystic Ovary Syndrome (PCOS)

PCOS is a kind of chronic anovulation caused by inappropriate estrogen feedback to the hypothalamus-pituitary system. It is characterized by bilaterally polycystic ovaries and a complex of symptoms consisting of menstrual disorders (amenorrhea, oligomenorrhea, or dysfunctional uterine bleeding), infertility, hirsutism, obesity, and a miscellany of underlying biochemical irregularities.

Treatment with clomiphene, traditional Chinese medicine, or gonadotropins is successful in about 70-80% of cases. Because of the risk of postoperative adhesions, ovarian wedge resection is used only when conservative treatment has failed. Generally the prognosis for PCOS is good, but in a few cases endometrial carcinoma may develop.

In traditional Chinese medicine, enlarged ovaries are seen as a consequence of water accumulating in the pelvic cavity where it transforms into phlegm, as a result of Kidney yang deficiency. Based on contemporary clinical observation, anovulation is attributed to Kidney deficiency. Some patients will also show signs of blood stasis. In general, PCOS involves Kidney deficiency, sometimes accompanied by constrained Liver qi, blood stasis, or phlegm.

Herbal treatment

STRATEGY: Tonify the Kidney yang, resolve the phlegm, and invigorate the blood.

Radix Rehmanniae Glutinosae Conquitae *(shu di huang)*..............12g
Radix Dioscoreae Oppositae *(shan yao)*................................12g
Rhizoma Polygonati *(huang jing)*.....................................12g
Herba Epimedii *(yin yang huo)*.......................................12g
Fructus Psoraleae Corylifoliae *(bu gu zhi)*..........................12g
Squama Manitis Pentadactylae *(chuan shan jia)*........................9g
Spina Gleditsiae Sinensis *(zao jiao ci)*.............................12g
Bulbus Fritillariae Cirrhosae *(chuan bei mu)*........................12g
Radix Angelicae Sinensis *(dang gui)*.................................12g
Semen Persicae *(tao ren)*..12g

MODIFICATIONS:

1. With signs of cold, add:
   Radix Lateralis Aconiti Carmichaeli Praeparata *(fu zi)*.............9g
   Cortex Cinnamomi Cassiae *(rou gui)*.................................3g

2. With constrained Liver qi, omit Spina Gleditsiae Sinensis *(zao jiao ci)* and Bulbus Fritillariae Cirrhosae *(chuan bei mu)*, and add:
   Cortex Moutan Radicis *(mu dan pi)*..................................9g
   Fructus Gardeniae Jasminoidis *(zhi zi)*............................12g
   Radix Bupleuri *(chai hu)*...6g
   Pericarpium Citri Reticulatae Viride *(qing pi)*.....................6g

ANALYSIS OF FORMULA: The purpose of this formula is to tonify the Kidneys. Radix Rehmanniae Glutinosae Conquitae *(shu di huang)*, Herba Epimedii *(yin yang huo),* and Fructus Psoraleae Corylifoliae *(bu gu zhi)* together have been shown to induce ovulation in cases of pubertal dysfunctional uterine bleeding. Rhizoma Polygonati *(huang jing)* serves to consolidate the yin so as to mitigate the warm properties of the other herbs.

MECHANISM OF ACTION: In one study, after treatment the patients' estrogen levels increased, and in some cases biphasic estrogen regulation was restored. Researchers found that these herbs act by regulating the LH receptors. It was therefore concluded that this formula has a definite effect in regulating ovarian function. Squama Manitis Pentadactylae *(chuan shan jia)*, Spina Gleditsiae Sinensis *(zao jiao ci),* and Bulbus Fritillariae Cirrhosae *(chuan bei mu)* can resolve the phlegm, that is, they may reverse the thickening of the ovarian capsule and the follicular atresia by antagonizing androgens.

Evidence shows that this formula will increase FSH and E_2 levels and thus reduce the LH/FSH and the T/E_2 ratios. Increased E_2 levels will act as positive feedback and thus cause ovulation. It seems that this formula acts not only on the ovary, but on the hypothalamus-pituitary system as well. In about 20% of cases, breast engorgement and elevated PRL levels were found; in those cases the formula was effective only when modified according to the pattern of constrained Liver qi. This verifies that elevated PRL levels and breast engorgement are indeed correlated with the traditional Chinese medical concept of constrained Liver qi.

EFFICACY: In one study, 133 patients were treated using this formula, of which 82.7% ovulated. Of the 76 infertile women, 36 became pregnant.

Acupuncture treatment

STRATEGY: Induce ovulation. The reader is referred to the section on inducing ovulation with acupuncture at the end of this chapter.

Hyperinsulinemia and Hyperandrogenism

Some chronic anovulatory cases manifest with signs and symptoms similar to PCOS, but with normal serum LH and elevated insulin and testosterone, particularly during the oral glucose tolerance test (OGTT). Insulin is one of the factors which may act synergistically with gonadotropin to make the ovarian theca and interstitial cells produce an excess of testosterone. No biomedical treatment has yet to achieve a satisfactory treatment for this syndrome.

In my own experience, when a patient with oligomenorrhea or amenorrhea complains of thirst and feeling warm, they will also have low estrogen and relatively high testosterone levels in the serum. From a traditional perspective, this means that there is yin deficiency, not heat excess. Patients often complain about acne or rough skin, and report intense thirst. We may therefore infer that this pattern of deficiency affects not only the Kidneys, but the Stomach and Lungs as well. One way of looking at it is that the thirst and feeling of warmth are related to the atrophy and thinness of the oral, respiratory, and digestive mucosa. Biomedically, this thinness is due to the decrease in serum estrogen and estrogen receptors.

Herbal treatment

STRATEGY: Replenish the yin of the Lungs, Stomach, and Kidneys in order to clear the internal heat and restore the reproductive functional balance.

Rhizoma Anemarrhenae Asphodeloidis *(zhi mu)* 12g
Cortex Phellodendri *(huang bai)* 12g
Radix Rehmanniae Glutinosae *(sheng di huang)* 18g
Tuber Ophiopogonis Japonici *(mai men dong)* 12g
Radix Trichosanthis Kirilowii *(tian hua fen)* 15g
Fructus Corni Officinalis *(shan zhu yu)*...............................12g
Herba Epimedii *(yin yang huo)* 12g

METHOD: Take daily as a decoction for three months. If no ovulation occurs, the same treatment in combination with clomiphene is recommended.

ANALYSIS OF FORMULA: Radix Rehmanniae Glutinosae *(sheng di huang)*, Tuber Ophiopogonis Japonici *(mai men dong)*, Fructus Corni Officinalis *(shan zhu yu)*, and Radix Trichosanthis Kirilowii *(tian hua fen)* together support the yin of the Lungs, Stomach, and Kidneys. Rhizoma Anemarrhenae Asphodeloidis *(zhi mu)* and Cortex Phellodendri *(huang bai)* clear internal heat and serve to protect the yin from injury due to excessive heat. Herba Epimedii *(yin yang huo)* is warm in nature and is used to mitigate the cold properties of the other herbs.

MECHANISM OF ACTION: The average patient does not respond to clomiphene prior to treatment with traditional Chinese medicine. This is because the high level of testosterone is caused by the elevated insulin level, rather than by the change in LH level. This formula can reduce the insulin level, and thereby induce the ovaries to produce less testosterone. Follicular growth will no longer be inhibited by testosterone. The level of estrogen will in turn increase, and either the follicles will develop normally, or the patient will at least become responsive to clomiphene.

EFFICACY: Patients suffering from hyperinsulinemia and hyperandrogenism show good results from this treatment, as evidenced by ovulation or pregnancy. It has also been shown that this herbal formula is effective in lowering elevated insulin and testosterone levels in rats.

Hypothalamic-Pituitary Amenorrhea

A woman who misses her period for more than six months and shows no sign of pregnancy can be said to have amenorrhea. If her serum gonadotropin level is low and her prolactin level normal, her condition is called hypothalamic-pituitary amenorrhea. Response to LRH test, which assesses gonadotropin secretion from the pituitary, is often decreased or delayed. The usual treatment is to attempt to induce ovulation with LHRH or HMG, or to prescribe a hormone replacement.

Traditional Chinese medicine has identified many factors which can cause amenorrhea: deficiency of the Kidneys, Liver/Kidney, or Spleen/Kidney deficiency, phlegm, blood stasis, qi and/or blood deficiency. Based on clinical observation, hypothalamic-pituitary amenorrhea is always related to Kidney and Spleen deficiency, sometimes complicated by blood stasis or phlegm.

Herbal treatment

STRATEGY: Tonify the Kidneys and the Spleen. Herbs that invigorate the blood, or that transform phlegm, are added when appropriate.

Radix Lateralis Aconiti Carmichaeli Praeparata *(fu zi)*....................9g
Cortex Cinnamomi Cassiae *(rou gui)*.......................................3g
Radix Rehmanniae Glutinosae Conquitae *(shu di huang)*...............12g
Rhizoma Polygonati *(huang jing)*...15g
Herba Epimedii *(yin yang huo)*...12g
Fructus Psoraleae Corylifoliae *(bu gu zhi)*...............................12g
Squama Manitis Pentadactylae *(chuan shan jia)*.........................9g
Semen Persicae *(tao ren)*..12g
Radix Angelicae Sinensis *(dang gui)*..9g
Spina Gleditsiae Sinensis *(zao jiao ci)*....................................12g

MODIFICATIONS:

With late ovulation, omit Radix Lateralis Aconiti Carmichaeli Praeparata *(fu zi)* and Cortex Cinnamomi Cassiae *(rou gui)*, and add:

Radix Codonopsitis Pilosulae *(dang shen)*................................12g
Rhizoma Atractylodis Macrocephalae *(bai zhu)*.........................12g

ANALYSIS OF FORMULA: The herbs in this formula are rather similar to those used in the treatment of PCOS. Herbs that tonify the Spleen and Kidneys are used along with Squama Manitis Pentadactylae *(chuan shan jia)* and Spina Gleditsiae Sinensis *(zao jiao ci)*, which transform phlegm and invigorate the blood. However, fewer herbs are used here than in the treatment of PCOS because the ovarian capsule is not as thick in hypothalamic-pituitary amenorrhea. Radix Angelicae Sinensis *(dang gui)* and Semen Persicae *(tao ren)* are used to invigorate the blood.

MECHANISM OF ACTION: The herbs in this formula have proven effective in increasing LH secretions from the pituitary in rats. Clinically, patients' response to the LRH test is increased or normalized.

EFFICACY: In one study, this treatment was 76% effective in restoring ovulation and menstruation in hypothalamic-pituitary amenorrhea patients. When the estrogen level was very low, estrogen was added to the treatment.

Galactorrhea-Amenorrhea Syndrome

Patients with no menses and who leak milk are usually infertile, show elevated prolactin levels, and have decreased libido. Causes other than pregnancy include pituitary tumors, hypothyroidism, PCOS with low central dopamine levels, drugs (e.g., chlorpromazine), chest wall trauma, and nipple stimulation. Elevated prolactin levels interfere with hypothalamic-pituitary-ovarian function to varying degrees, and thus this syndrome can manifest with different signs and symptoms.

Bromocriptine (Parlodel, Pravidel), a dopamine agonist, lowers serum prolactin, stops galactorrhea, and helps restore menses in patients affected by this syndrome. If the serum prolactin level is not elevated, or if PCOS is present, herbal treatment is indicated. If the prolactin level is elevated and there is no PCOS, bromocriptine is the drug of choice; herbal formulas can be used to make the patient more comfortable.

The breast is connected to the Liver channel, and the frequent presence of such symptoms as leakage of milk, headache, sensation of heat in the eyes with pressure, breast tenderness, thirst, amenorrhea, irritability, sensation of internal heat, red tongue or wiry pulse, are attributed in traditional Chinese medicine to Liver fire and Kidney and Liver yin deficiency.

Herbal treatment

Galactorrhea-Amenorrhea Syndrome Formula 1

STRATEGY: Facilitate the flow of Liver qi, clear the Liver fire, and replenish the Kidney and Liver yin.

Cortex Moutan Radicis *(mu dan pi)* 9g

Dry-fried Fructus Gardeniae Jasminoidis *(chao zhi zi)* 12g

Radix Bupleuri *(chai hu)* 6g

Pericarpium Citri Reticulatae Viride *(qing pi)* 6g

Radix Rehmanniae Glutinosae *(sheng di huang)* 18g

Rhizoma Polygonati *(huang jing)* 12g

Herba Epimedii *(yin yang huo)* 12g

Fructus Psoraleae Corylifoliae *(bu gu zhi)* 12g

Squama Manitis Pentadactylae *(chuan shan jia)* 9g

Radix Angelicae Sinensis *(dang gui)* 12g

METHOD: Take daily as a decoction for one to two months.

ANALYSIS OF FORMULA: Cortex Moutan Radicis *(mu dan pi)* and dry-fried Fructus Gardeniae Jasminoidis *(chao zhi zi)* clear Liver fire. Radix Bupleuri *(chai hu)* is used here to guide the actions of the other herbs to the Liver channel; it also promotes the free flow of qi in the Liver. Pericarpium Citri Reticulatae Viride *(qing pi)*, Squama Manitis Penta-dactylae *(chuan shan jia),* and Radix Angelicae Sinensis *(dang gui)* are effective in promoting the movement of qi and blood. Radix Rehmanniae Glutinosae *(sheng di huang),* Herba Epimedii *(yin yang huo),* Rhizoma Polygonati *(huang jing),* and Fructus Psoraleae Corylifoliae *(bu gu zhi)* all tonify the Kidneys. The combination of Radix Rehmanniae Glutinosae *(sheng di huang)* and Radix Angelicae Sinensis *(dang gui)* is especially effective in replenishing the Liver yin.

EFFICACY: This formula has proven effective in treating cases of PCOS with elevated prolactin levels. After treatment the prolactin levels returned to normal and ovulation resumed. It has also been effective in treating galactorrhea.

Galactorrhea-Amenorrhea Syndrome Formula 2

Fructus Hordei Vulgaris Germinatus Recens *(sheng mai ya)* 200g

METHOD: Prepare as a tea and drink over the course of the entire day.

ANALYSIS OF FORMULA: In the traditional Chinese literature, Fructus Hordei Vulgaris Germinatus Recens *(sheng mai ya)* is said to be quite effective in restraining lactation to be used postpartum.

MECHANISM OF ACTION: In experiments with rats, Fructus Hordei Vulgaris Germinatus Recens *(sheng mai ya)* lowered elevated prolactin levels back to normal.

Premature Ovarian Failure and Gonadotropin-Resistant Ovary Syndrome

This syndrome belongs to the category of hypergonadotropic amenorrheas. Its differential diagnosis is based on pathological study of the ovaries. There is premature ovarian failure when there are no follicles left and the patient is less than 35 years of age. In the gonadotropin-resistant ovary syndrome, follicles are present but do not develop. Destruction of FSH receptors as the result of an autoimmune disorder has been suggested as a possible cause. Because of high gonadotropin and low estrogen levels, patients experience symptoms similar to those of menopause: atrophy of the reproductive organs (including the breasts), hot flashes, irritability, and mood changes, among others. Except for replacement estrogen and progesterone, there are no available treatments in biomedicine.

Examination may reveal hot flashes, internal sensations of heat, thirst, irritability, lower back pain, dryness of the eyes, mouth, and vagina, a red tongue, and a rapid, fine pulse. This symptom complex relates to Kidney yin deficiency leading to internal heat. The loss of yin in turn causes a reduction in qi, as the yin serves as the material basis for the growth and transformation represented by the qi and yang. The patient will tend to feel tired, and will frequently catch cold.

Herbal treatment

STRATEGY: Replenish the Kidney yin, clear internal heat, and invigorate the blood.

Rhizoma Anemarrhenae Asphodeloidis *(zhi mu)* 12g
Cortex Phellodendri *(huang bai)* 12g
Radix Rehmanniae Glutinosae *(sheng di huang)* 15g
Plastrum Testudinis *(gui ban)*. 12g
Carapax Amydae Sinensis *(bie jia)* 12g
Fructus Ligustri Lucidi *(nu zhen zi)*. 12g
Herba Epimedii *(yin yang huo)* 12g
Fructus Psoraleae Corylifoliae *(bu gu zhi)* 12g
Radix Paeoniae Rubrae *(chi shao)* 12g
Semen Persicae *(tao ren)* 12g
Radix Angelicae Sinensis *(dang gui)*. 12g
Radix Pseudostellariae Heterophyllae *(tai zi shen)* 12g

METHOD: Take daily as a decoction, adding large doses of diethylstilbe-strol (0.5 to 1mg per day) during the last 20 days of each menstrual cycle. The course of treatment is one to two years.

MODIFICATION:

With agitation and unreasonable temper, add:

Cortex Moutan Radicis *(mu dan pi)*. 9g
Fructus Gardeniae Jasminoidis *(zhi zi)*. 12g

ANALYSIS OF FORMULA: Radix Rehmanniae Glutinosae *(sheng di huang)*, Cortex Phellodendri *(huang bai)*, Carapax Amydae Sinensis *(bie jia)*, and Fructus Ligustri Lucidi *(nu zhen zi)* are essential for replenishing the Kidney yin. Rhizoma Anemarrhenae Asphodeloidis *(zhi mu)* and Cortex Phellodendri *(huang bai)* clear internal heat in order to protect the Kidney yin from consumption. Herba Epimedii *(yin yang huo)* and Fructus Psoraleae Corylifoliae *(bu gu zhi)* are used to tonify the Kidneys while mitigating the cold properties of the other herbs. Radix Pseudostellariae Heterophyllae *(tai zi shen)* is useful in cases of mild qi deficiency. In chronic gynecological diseases, herbs which invigorate the blood are often used despite the absence of visible signs of blood stasis. One reason for this is that the pelvis, especially those aspects related to gynecological functions, is closely related to the Liver (and also the Kidneys). As the Liver is the reservoir of blood, Liver constraint (or any problem affecting the pelvis) can cause qi stagnation and blood stasis. Another reason is that chronic gynecological disorders usually involve relatively intense qi deficiency. This retards the flow of blood, making the woman more likely to develop blood stasis. Finally, especially with chronic problems, during the early stages of blood stasis it is common for there to be no visible signs. That is why Radix Paeoniae Rubrae *(chi shao)*, Semen Persicae *(tao ren)*, and Radix Angelicae Sinensis *(dang gui)* are included in this formula.

MECHANISM OF ACTION: Following the course of herbal treatment, the patient's estrogen level rises slightly. This results in an improvement in the dryness of the mouth, eyes, and vagina, as well as the hot flashes and sensations of heat. The patient feels calmer and more comfortable, and is less likely to catch cold. If the herbal treatment is administered in combination with estrogen therapy, the patient will experience relief of all her symptoms. Ovulation and even pregnancy may occur, especially in the case of gonadotropin-resistant ovary syndrome. This treatment works mostly by regulating the neuroendocrine immune system.

EFFICACY: In one study, three patients suffering from premature ovarian failure, and three from gonadotropin-resistant ovary syndrome, were treated with a combination of herbal and hormone therapy. After one to two years of treatment, two became pregnant and the other four showed firm evidence of ovulation.

Inducing Ovulation with Acupuncture

In the traditional literature the reproductive function is closely related to the Kidneys, Liver, and Spleen and their corresponding channels, as well as the Governing and Conception vessels. The main points for treating reproductive dysfunctions are therefore located on one of these five channels. While other points on other channels may also affect these functions, none is as important as these. In recent decades, studies of treatments given to induce ovulation have shown efficacy rates of around 50%.

Twenty-five percent of women treated for infertility associated with anovulation have become pregnant. Acupuncture is especially effective when infertility is caused by a hypothalamic disorder.

Acupuncture treatment

CV-3 *(zhong ji)*
CV-4 *(guan yuan)*
M-CA-18 *(zi gong xue)*[1]
SP-6 *(san yin jiao)*

METHOD: Needles inserted into the lower abdomen should go deep into the fascia, with the sensation extending into the vulva. Provide mild to moderate stimulation for 30 minutes for three consecutive days, starting on the 14th day after the last day of menses. If there are no menses, treatment is started immediately. Electro-stimulation is used, with a frequency of three Hertz, at a mild and comfortable intensity.

ANALYSIS OF TREATMENT: CV-3 *(zhong ji)* is the main point on the Conception vessel for regulating the reproductive functions. It is also a confluent point of the Kidney, Liver, and Spleen channels. CV-4 *(guan yuan)* is an important point for urogenital disorders. In the literature, M-CA-18 *(zi gong xue)* is described as a unique point for treating infertility. SP-6 *(san yin jiao)* is essential in treating all kinds of gynecological disorders because of its regulatory action on the Kidney, Liver, and Spleen channels.

MECHANISM OF ACTION: The general role of acupuncture is to promote the flow of qi and blood within the channels. However, not all patients have the same results with acupuncture. Studies indicate that inhibition of the sympathetic nervous system after acupuncture is a good indicator of the potential success of ovulation induction. This can be ascertained by using the hand temperature-change test. Points LI-4 *(he gu)* and PC-6 *(nei guan)* are needled for 30 minutes while the patient's hand temperature is monitored. If the hand temperature rises after treatment, the sympathetic nervous system is inhibited and the serum-endorphin level has been lowered. Such a patient is a good candidate for acupuncture. Studies also show that patients who have a low pulsatile frequency of LH and FSH experience, after treatment, an increase in gonadotropin pulsatile frequency, causing ovulation. These results suggest that acupuncture plays a central neuro-endocrinal function in inducing ovulation. Patients with high central opioid levels, as shown by the naloxone test, obtain better results than those with low central opioid levels. In these studies, peripheral estradiol levels match central opioid levels, thus serum estradiol levels may be taken to infer the activity of central-endorphin. The tone of the sympathetic nervous system is directly related to central opioid levels.

INDICATIONS: Anovulatory cases of pubertal dysfunctional uterine bleeding, hypothalamic-pituitary disorders, amenorrhea, PCOS with adequate estrogen levels. The ideal candidate should have a normal estrogen level, low gonadotropin frequency, and a positive response to the hand temperature-change test.

EFFICACY: Fifty to 60% of anovulatory patients ovulate after acupuncture. If patients are screened for the criteria described above, the success rate may be as high as 80%.

Endnote

1. This point is located 3 units lateral to CV-3 *(zhong ji)*.

Non-Anovulatory Menstrual Disorders

Luteal Phase Deficiency (LPD)

WHEN THE CORPUS luteum does not produce progesterone in sufficient amounts for two consecutive cycles, luteal phase deficiency is indicated. It is a known cause of infertility and is commonly associated with habitual miscarriage. Short periods or an atypical BBT are not sufficient diagnostic criteria for LPD. Even multiple blood progesterone assays during the luteal phase do not permit a definite diagnosis. Sometimes inadequate endometrial progesterone receptors do not permit the normal growth of the secretory endometrium. It has recently been suggested to perform an endometrial biopsy eight days after the BBT rise for two consecutive cycles. If the endometrium is two days out of phase on both cycles, then the diagnosis can be made. Sometimes LPD develops as a result of endometriosis.

LPD is often accompanied by polymenorrhea (bleeding between periods), habitual miscarriage, or infertility. Patients complain of low back pain, intolerance of cold, and fatigue; or they may experience irritability, breast tenderness, thirst, a feeling of internal heat, and dry eyes with a sensation of heat. The traditional pattern diagnosis would accordingly be Kidney yang deficiency, or Liver and Kidney yin deficiency, respectively.

Herbal treatment

Luteal Phase Deficiency Formula 1

STRATEGY: Tonify the Kidneys and invigorate the blood.

Radix Rehmanniae Glutinosae Conquitae *(shu di huang)* 12g

Plastrum Testudinis *(gui ban)* 12g

Rhizoma Atractylodis Macrocephalae *(bai zhu)* 10g

Radix Dipsaci Asperi *(xu duan)* 10g

Herba Cistanches *(rou cong rong)* 10g

Dry-fried Fructus Sophorae Japonicae *(chao huai hua)* 10g

Radix Angelicae Sinensis *(dang gui)* 10g

Fructus Psoraleae Corylifoliae *(bu gu zhi)* 12g

Semen Cuscutae Chinensis *(tu si zi)* 12g

METHOD: Take daily as a decoction for three months. NOTE: In the classical literature, Plastrum Testudinis *(gui ban)* is said to be contraindicated during pregnancy. Although this has not been verified in modern practice, more conservative practitioners may choose to substitute Fructus Ligustri Lucidi *(nu zhen zi)* and Tuber Ophiopogonis Japonici *(mai men dong)* for this ingredient.

MODIFICATIONS:

1. With Kidney yin deficiency, add:
   Fructus Ligustri Lucidi *(nu zhen zi)* 12g
   Herba Ecliptae Prostratae *(han lian cao)* 12g

2. With Kidney yang deficiency, add:
   Radix Morindae Officinalis *(ba ji tian)* 12g
   Radix Astragali Membranacei *(huang qi)* 12g

ANALYSIS OF FORMULA: Radix Rehmanniae Glutinosae Conquitae *(shu di huang)* and Plastrum Testudinis *(gui ban)* replenish the Kidney yin. Radix Dipsaci Asperi *(xu duan)*, Herba Cistanches *(rou cong rong)*, Semen Cuscutae Chinensis *(tu si zi),* and Fructus Psoraleae Corylifoliae *(bu gu zhi)* all tonify the Kidney yang, but are not so hot as to injure the yin. (It is always the rule to balance the yin and the yang.) When the patient tends toward yin deficiency, Fructus Ligustri Lucidi *(nu zhen zi)* and Herba Ecliptae Prostratae *(han lian cao)* are added to enrich and moisten. Radix Morindae Officinalis *(ba ji tian)* is used when the Kidney yang needs tonification, and in this case Radix Astragali Membranacei *(huang qi)* is a useful adjunct for increasing qi. Radix Angelicae Sinensis *(dang gui)* and dry-fried Fructus Sophorae Japonicae *(chao huai hua)* invigorate the blood and remove blood stasis, which benefits the local blood circulation and improves ovarian function.

MECHANISM OF ACTION: In the course of the herbal treatment, symptoms such as fatigue, low back pain, and thirst are relieved, and the BBT and serum progesterone return to normal. In experimental animals and in vitro, herbs which tonify the Kidneys can increase LH secretions and can also increase the progesterone contents in the corpus luteum of pseudopregnant rats.

EFFICACY: Studies have shown that 60-70% of women with LPD benefit from this formula after two to four months. When treating infertility due to LPD, 25-30% percent became pregnant within six months. In addition, continuing treatment throughout the pregnancy helps prevent miscarriage.

Luteal Phase Deficiency Formula 2

STRATEGY: Replenish the Kidney and Liver yin and clear the Liver fire to smooth the menstrual cycle.

Cortex Moutan Radicis *(mu dan pi)* 9g
Radix Scutellariae Baicalensis *(huang qin)* 15g

Radix Bupleuri *(chai hu)* 9g

Fructus Lycii *(gou qi zi)* 12g

Radix Rehmanniae Glutinosae *(sheng di huang)* 12g

Radix Paeoniae Lactiflorae *(bai shao)* 12g

Radix Angelicae Sinensis *(dang gui)* 12g

Fructus Corni Officinalis *(shan zhu yu)* 9g

Herba Epimedii *(yin yang huo)* 12g

Fructus Psoraleae Corylifoliae *(bu gu zhi)* 12g

Rhizoma Cyperi Rotundi *(xiang fu)* 12g

Sclerotium Poriae Cocos Rubrae *(chi fu ling)* 12g

METHOD: Take daily as a decoction for three months.

MODIFICATION:

With breast tenderness, add:

Tuber Curcumae *(yu jin)* 9g

Fructus Meliae Toosendan *(chuan lian zi)* 12g

Pericarpium Citri Reticulatae Viride *(qing pi)* 6g

ANALYSIS OF FORMULA: Radix Rehmanniae Glutinosae *(sheng di huang)*, Radix Paeoniae Lactiflorae *(bai shao)*, Fructus Corni Officinalis *(shan zhu yu)*, and Fructus Lycii *(gou qi zi)* together replenish both the Liver and Kidney yin. Herba Epimedii *(yin yang huo)* and Fructus Psoraleae Corylifoliae *(bu gu zhi)* are yang tonics which serve as a counterweight to the yin-tonifying herbs. Cortex Moutan Radicis *(mu dan pi)*, Radix Scutellariae Baicalensis *(huang qin)*, Radix Bupleuri *(chai hu)*, and Rhizoma Cyperi Rotundi *(xiang fu)* promote the smooth flow of Liver qi, clear Liver fire, and ease irritability. Sclerotium Poriae Cocos Rubrae *(chi fu ling)* gently drains internal heat through the urine. Tuber Curcumae *(yu jin)*, Fructus Meliae Toosendan *(chuan lian zi)*, and Pericarpium Citri Reticulatae Viride *(qing pi)* are especially effective in cases of Liver obstruction. Since the breasts are related to the Liver, these herbs are added when the breasts are tender.

MECHANISM OF ACTION: When LDP is accompanied by an imbalance in the Liver and Kidneys (breast tenderness, irritability, among other symptoms), the blood prolactin level may be slightly elevated. The herbs in this formula can alleviate the symptoms and help restore the prolactin to normal levels, which will enable the corpus luteum to produce more progesterone.

EFFICACY: Studies have shown that 70-80% of patients experience relief, and about one-third of patients treated for infertility become pregnant, within six to twelve months of treatment.

Functional Dysmenorrhea

Functional (primary) dysmenorrhea is intrinsic, idiopathic, painful menstruation that is not causally related to any identifiable gynecological disorder. It usually disappears after the first delivery. Painful cramps, corresponding with uterine contractions, usually occur with the onset of bleeding and last between a few hours and one to two days. Functional dysmenorrhea is accompanied by nausea in 50% of patients, with vomiting in 25%, and with frequent bowel movements in 35%.[1] In some cases the pain is relieved after expulsion of a membranous cast from the uterine cavity. When this happens it is referred to as "membranous" dysmenorrhea. Absorption of prostaglandins into the uterine circulation at the time of the endometrial breakdown is probably a cause of all the complaints. Non-steroidal anti-inflammatory drugs, aspirin, indomethacin, and other active inhibitors of prostaglandin synthesis are all usually effective in relieving the above symptoms.

According to traditional Chinese medicine, dysmenorrhea may be caused by qi stagnation or blood stasis or by exogenous cold lodging in the Womb. The usual picture is one of a combination of these patterns. Occasionally, Kidney deficiency may also be present. Patients complain of lower abdominal pain, cold, nausea, vomiting, and a sensation of being weighed down. They may see darker menstrual blood when pain is present.

Herbal treatment

Functional Dysmenorrhea Formula 1

STRATEGY: Promoting the local circulation of qi and blood is primary. Adjunctively, warming the Womb will help not only in relieving the cold sensation, but also in enhancing the flow of qi and blood.

Pollen Typhae *(pu huang)* 12g
Excrementum Trogopterori seu Pteromi *(wu ling zhi)* 12g
Radix Angelicae Sinensis *(dang gui)* 9g
Radix Salviae Miltiorrhizae *(dan shen)* 12g
Cortex Cinnamomi Cassiae *(rou gui)* 3g

METHOD: Take daily as a decoction starting two to five days before the menses, and continue until two or three days after the usual time of discomfort.

ANALYSIS OF FORMULA: Pollen Typhae *(pu huang)*, Excrementum Trogopterori seu Pteromi *(wu ling zhi)*, and Radix Salviae Miltiorrhizae *(dan shen)* invigorate the blood and remove stasis. The action of Cortex Cinnamomi Cassiae *(rou gui)* is to move the blood by warming. Radix Angelicae Sinensis *(dang gui)* is warm in nature and has the mild property of enhancing the flow of blood. Moreover, it is often used in gynecology to guide other herbs into the Womb. This herb is *not* recommended, however, in cases of significant heat.

MECHANISM OF ACTION: This formula has been shown to reduce prostaglandin F_{2a} levels in the endometrium and in the menstrual fluid of patients with functional dysmenorrhea. This action leads to reduced uterine hypertonic contractions. The menstrual blood was also observed to regain a bright color and a thin viscosity, which corroborates the traditional diagnosis of blood stasis.

EFFICACY: In one study of 198 cases with functional dysmenorrhea, 87.4% experienced relief from pain after one to three courses of treatment. An 18-month follow-up of 71 women showed that 77.5% had been cured.

Functional Dysmenorrhea Formula 2

This formula is especially well-suited for "membranous" dysmenorrhea.

STRATEGY: Promote the flow of qi and blood and remove blood stasis.

Pollen Typhae *(pu huang)* 15g
Excrementum Trogopterori seu Pteromi *(wu ling zhi)* 12g
Fructus Crataegi *(shan zha)* 12g
Pericarpium Citri Reticulatae Viride *(qing pi)* 4.5g
Sanguis Draconis *(xue jie)* 6g

MODIFICATIONS:

1. With internal heat, add:
   Herba cum Radice Patriniae *(bai jiang cao)* 30g
   Cooked Radix et Rhizoma Rhei *(zhi da huang)* 6g

2. With internal cold, add:
   Fructus Foeniculi Vulgaris *(xiao hui xiang)* 9g
   Quick-fried Rhizoma Zingiberis Officinalis *(pao jiang)* 3g

ANALYSIS OF FORMULA: Pollen Typhae *(pu huang)*, Excrementum Trogopterori seu Pteromi *(wu ling zhi)*, Fructus Crataegi *(shan zha)*, and Sanguis Draconis *(xue jie)* make a good combination for invigorating the blood and removing blood stasis. This combination has the advantage of not being cold, since cold often leads to pain. Pericarpium Citri Reticulatae Viride *(qing pi)* is used to promote the circulation of qi; it is a good idea to add herbs of this type when dealing with blood stasis, so that the qi can help move the blood. Herba cum Radice Patriniae *(bai jiang cao)* is used to reduce internal heat in the lower abdomen. Radix et Rhizoma Rhei *(da huang)*, when cooked, has the primary function of removing blood stasis and clearing heat; its purgative and detoxifying properties are less prominent. Fructus Foeniculi Vulgaris *(xiao hui xiang)* and quick-fried Rhizoma Zingiberis Officinalis *(pao jiang)* are warm in nature and are used to dispel cold from the lower abdomen and to regulate the flow of qi in the pelvic cavity. Fresh ginger, upon cooking, loses its exterior-releasing properties; it warms the lower abdomen, helps the circulation of blood, and indirectly assists in the production of blood.

MECHANISM OF ACTION: The herbs which encourage the circulation of blood in this formula have been shown to reduce high blood viscosity in dysmenorrhea patients. High blood viscosity is caused by elevated endometrial prostaglandin levels, and is associated with uterine spasms and thus dysmenorrhea. Using the formula, premenstrual estradiol levels were lowered. This may help control local prostaglandin levels and thus regulate the endometrium.

EFFICACY: In one study of 30 patients treated for "membranous" dysmenorrhea, relief from pain was achieved after three menstrual cycles in 87% of cases.

Acupuncture treatment

Method 1

SP-6 *(san yin jiao)*
SP-10 *(xue hai)*
CV-4 *(guan yuan)*

METHOD: Retain needles 30 minutes daily from one or two days before, and until the second day after, the onset of menses. In cases of cold, better results can be obtained by using moxa at CV-4 *(guan yuan)*.

EXPLANATION OF POINTS: SP-6 *(san yin jiao)* is a point of intersection for the Liver, Kidney, and Spleen channels, and is an important point in treating all kinds of gynecological disorders. It is used universally in the same way as Radix Angelicae Sinensis *(dang gui)* is used in herbal treatments. SP-10 *(xue hai)* is a special point for dispelling blood stasis. CV-4 *(guan yuan)* helps the circulation of qi and blood in the Conception vessel, which is closely associated with the Womb. Acupuncture has the effect of increasing serum beta-endorphin levels.

Method 2

Ear Acupuncture:

Uterus
Kidney
Ovary

METHOD: Secure magnetized pellets on the ear points. The pellets should be pressed for two minutes five times daily, but hourly on the first day of menstruation.

EXPLANATION OF POINTS: Ear point stimulation is a simple way to ease pain and cause the cervix to loosen and relax.

Method 3

Implant a 1cm (0.4 inch) piece of sterile absorbable suture (catgut), size "0", into point SP-6 *(san yin jiao)* at the usual needling depth, two to three days before the period. Repeat every three months.

EXPLANATION: Implanting catgut provides constant stimulation of the acupuncture point. This method should be reserved for recalcitrant cases that do not respond to other methods.

EFFICACY: In one study, about 70% of patients thus treated benefitted from the procedure.

Asherman's Syndrome

Asherman's syndrome refers to amenorrhea or hypomenorrhea with cyclic lower abdominal pain following destruction or loss of the endometrium. Its usual causes are overzealous curettage and severe intrauterine infection, with resulting scarification and multiple synechiae (adhesions). These interfere with normal menstrual flow and cause cramps. The usual treatment is to loosen the adhesions with another curettage and insert a ring-type IUD for three months to prevent new synechiae from forming. Estrogen therapy may be given at the same time. The treatment outcome may be further improved by combining the above with herbal therapy.

From a traditional Chinese medical perspective, this situation after curretage or infection results in injury to the vessels of the Womb, which causes blood stasis in the Womb; this prevents the normal flow of menstrual fluid. Such patients will always show blue spots on their tongue. Blood stasis is thus the main feature of Asherman's syndrome.

Herbal treatment

STRATEGY: Dispel the stasis and unblock the menstruation.

Radix Angelicae Sinensis *(dang gui)* 15g
Radix Paeoniae Rubrae *(chi shao)* 12g
Semen Persicae *(tao ren)* 15g
Radix Ligustici Chuanxiong *(chuan xiong)* 12g
Sanguis Draconis *(xue jie)* 6g
Flos Carthami Tinctorii *(hong hua)* 9g
Radix et Caulis Jixueteng *(ji xue teng)* 15g
Herba Epimedii *(yin yang huo)* 12g

METHOD: Take daily as a decoction for three cycles.

ANALYSIS OF FORMULA: All of the herbs in this formula, except Herba Epimedii *(yin yang huo)*, invigorate the blood in the Womb, guided by Radix Angelicae Sinensis *(dang gui)*. The menses can then flow easily. Herba Epimedii *(yin yang huo)* helps restore function to the Kidneys after chronic impairment. The Kidneys must be strong or else the adhesions will have a tendency to recur.

MECHANISM OF ACTION: In animal experiments, herbs that invigorate the blood have three proven effects. First, they reduce vascular permeability and reduce local edema for improved local circulation. Second, they increase monocyte and macrophage activity and thus permit better phagocytosis of dead tissues and foreign bodies to facilitate endometrial restoration. Herba Epimedii *(yin yang huo)* reinforces that effect. Third, they suppress the proliferation of fibroblasts and accelerate the degradation of collagen, thus leaving less opportunity for endometrial adhesions.

EFFICACY: IUD and herbal treatments combined have been shown to yield better results than the IUD treatment alone. In mild cases, combination treatment offers an excellent prognosis.

Menorrhagia

Menorrhagia is defined as cyclic menstrual bleeding in excessive amounts (greater than 80ml per cycle) with typical biphasic BBT and normal cycle length. It is commonly encountered in multiparous women and after tubal ligation, IUD insertion, or abortion by curettage. It is also a common symptom of uterine myoma, endometrial polyps, and adenomyosis, among other disorders. There do not appear to be any systemic causes, as cyclic hormonal profiles show normal values. The main underlying problem from a biomedical perspective appears to be prostaglandin disorders. Drugs that inhibit prostaglandin synthesis, such as indomethacin, are effective in reducing blood loss in some cases.

In Chinese medicine, menorrhagia is viewed as injury to the Conception and Penetrating vessels, which are closely linked to the Womb. The injury in such cases is associated with giving birth, curettage, IUD insertion, and other factors. The resulting blood stasis causes the blood to seek a pathway outside of its normal vessels and extravasate, with the resulting hemorrhage. The loss of blood may in turn deplete the yin and lead to heat from deficiency. This can have the effect of depleting the qi, and the condition may continue to worsen in a vicious cycle. The menstrual fluid, besides being abundant, may also be dark with clots. Patients may complain of premenstrual irritability, thirst, a sensation of internal heat, and constipation, and there may be blue spots on the tongue and purpura. If the qi is deficient, there will be pallor, fatigue, and a swollen tongue.

Herbal treatment

Safe Womb (gong tai)

STRATEGY: Dispel the blood stasis and replenish the qi and the yin.

Radix Rubiae Cordifoliae *(qian cao gen)* 12g

Fructus Sophorae Japonicae Immaturus *(huai hua mi)*.................. 12g

Pollen Typhae *(pu huang)* 12g

Radix Codonopsitis Pilosulae *(dang shen)* 12g

Rhizoma Atractylodis Macrocephalae *(bai zhu)* 6g

Rhizoma Cimicifugae *(sheng ma)* 9g

Radix Rehmanniae Glutinosae *(sheng di huang)* 12g

Radix Paeoniae Lactiflorae *(bai shao)* 9g

Fructus Ligustri Lucidi *(nu zhen zi)*....................................... 12g

Fructus Crataegi *(shan zha)*... 12g

Herba Ecliptae Prostratae *(han lian cao)*.................................. 12g

Herba seu Radix Cirsii Japonici *(da ji)*.................................... 12g

Herba Cephalanoplos Segeti *(xiao ji)* 12g

METHOD: Take daily as a decoction from seven days prior to menstruation until the end of bleeding, for three cycles. This formula has been approved by the Chinese Ministry of Public Health to be sold as a prepared medicine in tea form.

ANALYSIS OF FORMULA: Radix Rubiae Cordifoliae *(qian cao gen)*, Fructus Sophorae Japonicae Immaturus *(huai hua mi)*, Pollen Typhae *(pu huang)*, Fructus Crataegi *(shan zha)*, Herba seu Radix Cirsii Japonici *(da ji)*, and Herba Cephalanoplos Segeti *(xiao ji)* have cool properties; they invigorate the blood and dispel blood stasis. Radix Rehmanniae Glutinosae *(sheng di huang)*, Radix Paeoniae Lactiflorae *(bai shao)*, Herba Ecliptae Prostratae *(han lian cao)*, and Fructus Ligustri Lucidi *(nu zhen zi)* replenish the yin, reduce internal heat, and stop bleeding. Radix Codonopsitis Pilosulae *(dang shen)*, Rhizoma Atractylodis Macrocephalae *(bai zhu)*, and Rhizoma Cimicifugae *(sheng ma)* are essential in the treatment of qi deficiency, and do not injure the yin.

MECHANISM OF ACTION: Scientific data show that local prostaglandins are better regulated after treatment. Thromboxane B_2 and fibrinogen degradation product levels return to normal in the endometrium and menstrual fluids. Local prostaglandin E_2 values are raised to normal levels in patients with yin deficiency, while they are lowered to normal levels in patients with qi deficiency. This formula appears to reduce blood viscosity and strengthen clotting where blood vessels are ruptured. It also regulates the uterine and vascular muscular tone, as shown by in vitro tests. This formula would appear to act on coagulation, on fibrinolysis, and on the muscular tone via prostaglandins.

EFFICACY: In a study of 352 patients treated with this formula, 85% were cured or showed significant improvement.

Uterine Bleeding During Ovulation

Uterine bleeding during ovulation consists of slight bleeding in mid-cycle, around the time of ovulation, without any pathological changes in the endometrium. Its cause is probably a brief fall in the estrogen level just after follicular rupture. Administering a small dose of estrogen does not produce significant results, and a large dose will inhibit ovulation.

The traditional view of the menstrual cycle is as follows. The Kidneys are more active just after menstruation in order to rebuild the lost yin. Some women will show Kidney yin deficiency immediately after their menses. The yin builds up during the first part of the cycle, since it will be needed to control the yang during ovulation. At the time of ovulation the yin energy yields to yang energy, which is then predominant. The insufficiency of yin prevents it from adequately controlling the yang, and heat and bleeding ensue.

Herbal treatment

STRATEGY: Replenish the Kidneys, especially their yin aspect, and strengthen the Conception and Penetrating vessels.

Radix Rehmanniae Glutinosae *(sheng di huang)* 18g

Radix Rehmanniae Glutinosae Conquitae *(shu di huang)* 12g

Radix Paeoniae Lactiflorae *(bai shao)* 12g

Calcined Concha Ostreae *(duan mu li)* 15g

Fructus Corni Officinalis *(shan zhu yu)* 12g

Fructus Ligustri Lucidi *(nu zhen zi)* 12g

Herba Ecliptae Prostratae *(han lian cao)* 30g

Charred Cacumen Biotae Orientalis *(ce bai ye tan)* 15g

Charred Nodus Nelumbinis Nuciferae Rhizomatis *(ou jie tan)* 15g

Os Sepiae seu Sepiellae *(hai piao xiao)* 12g

METHOD: To preserve its properties, Cacumen Biotae Orientalis *(ce bai ye)* should be fried until the outer part turns black and the inner part yellowish brown. Take daily as a decoction for 20 days from the onset of menses.

ANALYSIS OF FORMULA: Radix Rehmanniae Glutinosae *(sheng di huang)*, Radix Rehmanniae Glutinosae Conquitae *(shu di huang)*, Fructus Corni Officinalis *(shan zhu yu)*, and Fructus Ligustri Lucidi *(nu zhen zi)* replenish the Kidney yin in order to control the yang. Concha Ostreae *(mu li)* is a yin tonic. Uncooked, it is used to soften and disperse hard lumps. Calcined, it tonifies the Kidney yin, clears internal heat, and prevents the leakage of fluids. Herba Ecliptae Prostratae *(han lian cao)* not only tonifies the yin, but also clears internal heat. Cacumen Biotae Orientalis *(ce bai ye)* and Nodus Nelumbinis Nuciferae Rhizomatis *(ou jie)* are slightly cool in nature, and are effective in clearing heat. When charred, they also stop bleeding. Os Sepiae seu Sepiellae *(hai piao xiao)* is an astringent that is used to preserve the yin and stop the bleeding.

MECHANISM OF ACTION: No pharmacological research has been performed with this formula. The hemostatic effect may be due to a better development of the ovarian follicle during the proliferative phase.

EFFICACY: It has been shown that two-thirds of patients treated with this formula can expect bleeding during ovulation to stop within two to four months.

Premenstrual Syndrome

Most women experience minimal premenstrual discomfort, which does not hinder their daily activities. Twenty to forty percent of women feel one or more of a broad range of symptoms that persist for one or two weeks prior to menstruation, and subside or diminish abruptly at the onset of the menses. If symptoms are severe enough to disrupt a woman's life pattern or impel her to seek medical relief, her condition is called premenstrual syndrome. Symptoms differ among women but are fairly constant from one cycle to the next for the same individual. They may take the form of affective changes such as nervousness, agitation, irritability, or depression; neurological changes such as headache, vertigo, or aggravation of epilepsy; respiratory symptoms such as colds, hoarseness of the voice, aggravation of asthma; or internal disturbances such as abdominal bloating, edema, breast tenderness, palpitations, and a feeling of bearing down in the pelvis, among other symptoms. The underlying causes are obscure. Imbalance between estrogen and progesterone, excess of ADH or of aldosterone, hypoglycemia, psychogenic factors, and recently, disturbances in the interaction between central opioids and catecholamines, have been suggested as possible contributing factors. Biomedical treatment is palliative and nonspecific. Small doses of testosterone may help, and in severe cases inhibition of ovulation with oral contraceptives or progestin can bring complete relief.

This syndrome has been widely described by traditional doctors who view it as related to infertility. Basic causes focus on deficiency of the Liver and Kidney yin, and the obstruction of Liver qi. The latter cause is responsible for the symptoms of the breasts and chest, which are traversed by the Liver channel. Liver fire arising from yin deficiency usually causes emotional and neurological changes such as irritability, depression, or headache. And when the Spleen is overcontrolled by the Liver, water accumulates and transforms into phlegm, which then rises to the head and causes vertigo, dizziness, or edema.

Herbal treatment

STRATEGY: Promote the free-flow of Liver qi, clear the Liver fire, replenish the Kidney yin, strengthen the Spleen, and expel the water and phlegm to regulate the menstrual cycle.

Premenstrual Syndrome Formula 1: Liver qi stagnation

Radix Bupleuri *(chai hu)*...9g
Radix Angelicae Sinensis *(dang gui)*..9g
Radix Paeoniae Lactiflorae *(bai shao)*.....................................12g
Spica Prunellae Vulgaris *(xia ku cao)*......................................12g
Nidus Vespae *(lu feng fang)*...12g
Tuber Curcumae *(yu jin)*..9g
Rhizoma Cyperi Rotundi *(xiang fu)*..9g
Fructus Meliae Toosendan *(chuan lian zi)*...................................12g
Semen Vaccariae Segetalis *(wang bu liu xing)*..............................12g

METHOD: As a decoction, take daily after menses stop for three to six months.

ANALYSIS OF FORMULA: All of these herbs enhance the flow of the Liver qi and ameliorate such symptoms as breast tenderness, fullness in the chest, and the sensation of bearing down. Some of the herbs deserve special discussion. Liver qi constraint can lead to heat, and premenstrual syndrome is often accompanied by fibrocystic breasts. Spica Prunellae Vulgaris *(xia ku cao)* is used here for its ability to clear Liver heat and reduce nodules. Semen Vaccariae Segetalis *(wang bu liu xing)* enters the Liver and Stomach channels; it is commonly used to promote both menstruation and lactation. This is because these fluids depend on the proper functioning of the yang brightness channel. In modern China, Nidus Vespae *(lu feng fang)* is used as a potent substance which promotes the flow of qi in the Liver and eliminates nodules. It is one that I use regularly at this dosage in decoctions, and have never observed any side effects or toxicity.

Premenstrual Syndrome Formula 2: Liver fire

Radix Bupleuri *(chai hu)*...9g

Radix Angelicae Sinensis *(dang gui)* 9g
Cortex Moutan Radicis *(mu dan pi)* 6g
Dry-fried Fructus Gardeniae Jasminoidis *(chao zhi zi)* 12g
Spica Prunellae Vulgaris *(xia ku cao)* 12g
Radix Ligustici Chuanxiong *(chuan xiong)* 9g
Rhizoma Cyperi Rotundi *(xiang fu)* 9g
Flos Rosae Rugosae *(mei gui hua)* 6g

ANALYSIS OF FORMULA: Cortex Moutan Radicis *(mu dan pi)*, Fructus Gardeniae Jasminoidis *(zhi zi)*, and Spica Prunellae Vulgaris *(xia ku cao)* enter the Liver channel and clear fire from the Liver. Radix Bupleuri *(chai hu)*, Rhizoma Cyperi Rotundi *(xiang fu)*, and Flos Rosae Rugosae *(mei gui hua)* expedite the flow of Liver qi. Radix Angelicae Sinensis *(dang gui)* and Radix Ligustici Chuanxiong *(chuan xiong)* invigorate the blood, a function closely related to helping the free-flow of qi.

Premenstrual Syndrome Formula 3: phlegm obstruction

Rhizoma Coptidis *(huang lian)* 6g
Fructus Citri seu Ponciri Immaturus *(zhi shi)* 9g
Spica Prunellae Vulgaris *(xia ku cao)* 12g
Cooked Radix et Rhizoma Rhei *(zhi da huang)* 6g
Cinnabar-processed Sclerotium Poriae Cocos Pararadicis *(zhu fu shen)* . . 12g
Ginger-prepared Rhizoma Pinelliae Ternatae *(jiang ban xia)* 9g
Rhizoma Arisaematis *(tian nan xing)* 12g
Rhizoma Acori Graminei *(shi chang pu)* 12g
Radix Polygalae Tenuifoliae *(yuan zhi)* 9g
Ramulus cum Uncis Uncariae *(gou teng)* 12g

ANALYSIS OF FORMULA: Rhizoma Coptidis *(huang lian)*, Fructus Citri seu Ponciri Immaturus *(zhi shi)*, and Radix et Rhizoma Rhei *(da huang)* clear heat and remove phlegm from the Middle Burner. Although Radix et Rhizoma Rhei *(da huang)* is a purgative, when it is cooked it can clear heat and resolve phlegm in the Middle Burner without purging.[2] Rhizoma

Pinelliae Ternatae *(ban xia)* and Rhizoma Arisaematis *(tian nan xing)* resolve phlegm, and, in their prepared form, will not irritate the Stomach. Rhizoma Acori Graminei *(shi chang pu)* is used to resolve phlegm. The sedative function of Sclerotium Poriae Cocos Pararadicis *(fu shen)*, an herb that calms the spirit, is enhanced when processed with Cinnabaris *(zhu sha)*. Radix Polygalae Tenuifoliae *(yuan zhi)* and Ramulus cum Uncis Uncariae *(gou teng)* both act to calm the spirit, but the former also resolves phlegm, while the latter extinguishes Liver wind.

Premenstrual Syndrome Formula 4: Spleen deficiency

Radix Codonopsitis Pilosulae *(dang shen)* 12g
Rhizoma Atractylodis Macrocephalae *(bai zhu)* 9g
Cinnabar-processed Sclerotium Poriae Cocos Pararadicis *(zhu fu shen)* 12g
Sclerotium Polypori Umbellati *(zhu ling)* 12g
Rhizoma Alismatis Orientalis *(ze xie)* 12g
Semen Plantaginis *(che qian zi)* 12g
Radix Angelicae Sinensis *(dang gui)* 9g
Radix Ligustici Chuanxiong *(chuan xiong)* 9g
Spica Prunellae Vulgaris *(xia ku cao)* 12g
Radix Bupleuri *(chai hu)* 9g

METHOD: Starting at the end of menstruation, and for three cycles, take daily as a decoction for 20 days.

ANALYSIS OF FORMULA: Radix Codonopsitis Pilosulae *(dang shen)* and Rhizoma Atractylodis Macrocephalae *(bai zhu)* benefit the Spleen and drain water. Sclerotium Polypori Umbellati *(zhu ling)*, Rhizoma Alismatis Orientalis *(ze xie)*, and Semen Plantaginis *(che qian zi)* expel water without injuring the yin. Cinnabar-processed Sclerotium Poriae Cocos Pararadicis *(zhu fu shen)* helps calm the spirit. Radix Bupleuri *(chai hu)* and Spica Prunellae Vulgaris *(xia ku cao)* expedite the flow of Liver qi and clear Liver fire. Radix Angelicae Sinensis *(dang gui)* and Radix Ligustici Chuanxiong *(chuan xiong)* invigorate the blood and benefit the Liver.

MODIFICATIONS (applicable to all the formulas in this section):

1. With headache, add:
   Fructus Viticis *(man jing zi)* 9g
   Fructus Tribuli Terrestris *(bai ji li)* 12g

2. With depression, add:
   Honey-toasted Radix Glycyrrhizae Uralensis *(zhi gan cao)* 6g
   Semen Tritici Aestivi Levis *(fu xiao mai)* 12g
   Fructus Zizyphi Jujubae *(da zao)* 12g

3. With constipation, add:
   Radix Angelicae Sinensis *(dang gui)* 10g
   Radix Gentianae Longdancao *(long dan cao)* 5g
   Fructus Gardeniae Jasminoidis *(zhi zi)* 10g
   Rhizoma Coptidis *(huang lian)* 10g
   Cortex Phellodendri *(huang bai)* 10g
   Radix Scutellariae Baicalensis *(huang qin)* 10g
   Herba Aloes *(lu hui)* 5g
   Radix et Rhizoma Rhei *(da huang)* 5g
   Radix Aucklandiae Lappae *(mu xiang)* 1.5g
   Secretio Moschus *(she xiang)* 0.5g

This formula is called Tangkuei, Gentiana Longdancao and Aloe Pill *(dang gui long hui wan)* and is very useful in treating the constipation associated with Liver fire.

MECHANISM OF ACTION: It has been shown that not only are the symptoms relieved during the course of herbal treatment, but most BBT cycles are also restored to normal. This suggests a regulatory effect on the neuroendocrine reproductive system.

EFFICACY: In a study of 73 women treated with herbs for premenstrual syndrome, in which the treatment was adjusted according to individual needs, 46 were cured, 24 improved, and three did not respond to treatment. Among the 21 infertile women in the study, eight of them became pregnant.

Periodic (Menstrual) Migraine

Menstrual migraine is a severe headache associated with sensory and motor disturbances such as vomiting or dark spots in the visual field. It may persist even after menopause. The true cause is unknown, although abnormal levels of central neurotransmitters such as serotonin have been measured. Symptomatic treatment is routinely used, and Sumatriptan, a serotonin agonist, may relieve the headache.

In traditional Chinese medicine, menstrual migraine is divided into two types based on the symptoms. The first pattern is the Liver type, displaying signs of Liver yin deficiency and of Liver fire flaring upward, with feelings of internal heat, thirst, constipation, a hot sensation in the eyes, a unilateral headache covering the eye, temple, ear, and occipital area, nausea, and vomiting. The second pattern is the Stomach type and is caused by damp-heat in the Stomach channel, which disturbs the head as well. Such patients experience poor appetite and vomiting, and the headache covers the forehead and top of the head up to the occipital area. These patients typically present with a coated tongue, and may sometimes exhibit signs and symptoms of qi deficiency, such as fatigue, pallor, and fear of cold.

Acupuncture treatment

Ear acupuncture has proven to be most effective and free of side effects.

Method 1: Liver-type menstrual migraine

Occiput and/or Temple	Kidney
Eye	Shenmen
Liver	Stomach

METHOD: Locate the points on the ear by pressing for the most sensitive spot in their likely area. Secure magnetic pellets on one ear, five days before menstruation begins. Press the pellets with force for two minutes, five times a day. Alternate with the other ear after four days, and continue at that ear for another four days, or until the period is over.

EXPLANATION OF POINTS: The area affected by this type of headache is along the Gall Bladder channel. This channel is paired with the Liver, and the sensation of heat in the eyes also suggests Liver involvement. The thirst, constipation, and sensation of internal heat are evidence of yin deficiency, which leads to Liver fire. The ear points Liver, Eye, Occiput and/or Temple, and Kidney were chosen to address this aspect of the disorder. The ear point Shenmen was chosen for its sedative effect. The Stomach point was selected to prevent the Liver fire from injuring the Spleen, as expressed in the five-phase relationship, "wood controls earth."

Method 2: Stomach-type menstrual migraine

Forehead or Temple	Liver
Stomach	Bladder
Shenmen	

METHOD: Attach magnetic pellets in the same manner as described in the first method.

EXPLANATION OF POINTS: Dampness can easily reach the Spleen and Stomach channels. According to five-phase theory, the weaker the Spleen, the stronger the Liver. If there are Liver symptoms such as irritability, the Liver qi is probably predominant. In such cases, add the Liver point. The Bladder point is used to expel heat through urination.

MECHANISM OF ACTION: The ear is an area where all the channels meet, and it is in close proximity to the site of pain. This makes ear acupuncture a likely avenue for treatment based on improving cerebrovascular tone. When the pellets are pressed against the ear, local redness can be seen, an obvious sign of increased blood flow.

EFFICACY: In one study, 80-90% of patients experienced relief from their headache after one or two cycles of treatment.

Endnotes

1. Benson, R. C., *Current Obstetric & Gynecologic Diagnosis & Treatment.* Los Aptos, CA: Lange Medical Pulications, 1980, p. 114.

2. This usage, which is very effective clinically, goes back at least to the eighteenth century work *Thoroughly Revised Materia Medica (Ben cao cong xin)* by Wu Yi-Luo.

Complications
of Pregnancy

Viral Hepatitis

THE MANIFESTATIONS OF epidemic hepatitis (mainly types A or B) may be more severe when the disease occurs in advanced pregnancy. Acute yellow atrophy of the Liver may be fatal. Fetal abnormalities are increased about twofold if hepatitis develops during the first trimester of pregnancy. As with the nonpregnant patient, treatment is supportive. With good obstetrical care and nutrition, the maternal mortality rate is about the same as that of nonpregnant patients. Anesthetics, analgesics, and sedatives may be hepatotoxic. In order to prevent hemorrhage, vitamin K should be administered when the plasma prothrombin concentration is low.

In traditional Chinese medicine, jaundice during pregnancy is viewed as yang or yin jaundice caused by external toxins becoming entangled with fetal heat, and transforming into fire toxin within both mother and fetus. The fire toxin lodges in the Middle Burner where it disturbs the function of the Liver, Spleen, Gall Bladder, and Stomach. The bile no longer follows its proper pathway, which results in jaundice and yellow urine. Stagnation in the Middle Burner results in hypochondriac pain, fever, thirst, vomiting, nausea, poor appetite, and fatigue. Heat may cause the fire of the Liver to rise and produce wind and convulsions. If fire toxin enters the mother's blood, disseminated bleeding and petechiae will appear, and death may follow. If the disease becomes chronic, Liver deficiency may exhaust the Kidneys. Blood stasis sets in and the jaundice takes on a dark yellow appearance. This is called yin jaundice, which will not be discussed here.

Herbal treatment

STRATEGY: Clear the heat and relieve the toxicity in the Liver and Gall Bladder, and prevent miscarriage.

Herba Artemisiae Yinchenhao *(yin chen hao)* 30g
Herba Artemisiae Annuae *(qing hao)* 10g
Herba Lysimachiae *(jin qian cao)* 30g
Radix Astragali Membranacei *(huang qi)* 15g
Fructus Gardeniae Jasminoidis *(zhi zi)* 10g
Radix et Rhizoma Rhei *(da huang)* 3g
Radix Scutellariae Baicalensis *(huang qin)* 12g
Semen Cuscutae Chinensis *(tu si zi)* 10g
Fructus Hordei Vulgaris Germinatus Recens *(sheng mai ya)* 20g

MODIFICATIONS:

1. With severe heat, double the dosage of Radix Scutellariae Baicalensis *(huang qin)* and Herba Artemisiae Annuae *(qing hao)*.

2. With dampness, add:
   Sclerotium Polypori Umbellati *(zhu ling)* 12g
   Sclerotium Poriae Cocos *(fu ling)* 12g
   Semen Coicis Lachryma-jobi *(yi yi ren)* 12g

3. With hypochondriac pain, add:
   Tuber Curcumae *(yu jin)* 9g
   Fructus Meliae Toosendan *(chuan lian zi)* 12g

4. With abdominal distention, add:
Radix Aucklandiae Lappae *(mu xiang)* 3g
Cortex Magnoliae Officinalis *(hou po)*. 6g

5. With intractable, high fever, add:
Flos Lonicerae Japonicae *(jin yin hua)* 15g
Fructus Forsythiae Suspensae *(lian qiao)* 15g
Powdered Cornu Antelopis *(ling yang jiao)* 2g

6. With qi deficiency, increase the dosage of Radix Astragali
Membranacei *(huang qi)* to 30g, and add:
Radix Codonopsitis Pilosulae *(dang shen)* 15g

7. With a poor appetite, add:
Endothelium Corneum Gigeriae Galli *(ji nei jin)* 12g
Baked Fructus Oryzae Sativae Germinatus *(wei gu ya)*. 12g

8. With constipation, increase the dosage of Radix et
Rhizoma Rhei *(da huang)* to 6g.

ANALYSIS OF FORMULA: Herba Artemisiae Yinchenhao *(yin chen hao)*,
Herba Artemisiae Annuae *(qing hao)*, Herba Lysimachiae *(jin qian cao)*,
Fructus Gardeniae Jasminoidis *(zhi zi)*, and Radix Scutellariae Baicalensis
(huang qin) all clear excessive heat from the Liver. Herba Lysimachiae *(jin
qian cao)* also regulates the flow of bile. In addition, Radix Scutellariae
Baicalensis *(huang qin)* is effective in preventing miscarriage. Radix et
Rhizoma Rhei *(da huang)*, a strong purgative, eases the jaundice by
increasing the flow of bile. In order to mitigate the purgative action of
Radix et Rhizoma Rhei *(da huang)*, the deputies Radix Astragali
Membranacei *(huang qi)*, Radix Codonopsitis Pilosulae *(dang shen)*, and
Semen Cuscutae Chinensis *(tu si zi)* are added. These herbs also have a
rising nature, which thereby strengthens the Womb and prevents miscarriage. Sclerotium Polypori Umbellati *(zhu ling)*, Sclerotium Poriae Cocos
(fu ling), and Semen Coicis Lachryma-jobi *(yi yi ren)* clear heat through
diuresis. Tuber Curcumae *(yu jin)* and Fructus Meliae Toosendan *(chuan
lian zi)* are special herbs for Liver obstruction. Radix Aucklandiae Lappae
(mu xiang) and Cortex Magnoliae Officinalis *(hou po)* regulate the Intes-

tines and ease abdominal distention. Flos Lonicerae Japonicae *(jin yin hua)* and Fructus Forsythiae Suspensae *(lian qiao)* clear heat. Cornu Antelopis *(ling yang jiao),* in addition to clearing heat, also subdues the fire of the Liver and dispels internal wind. Endothelium Corneum Gigeriae Galli *(ji nei jin)* and baked Fructus Oryzae Sativae Germinatus *(wei gu ya)* eliminate food stagnation.

MECHANISM OF ACTION: This formula acts by reducing the elevated levels of glutamic pyruvic transaminase, thereby normalizing hepatic cellular function. Herba Artemisiae Yinchenhao *(yin chen hao)* has choleretic properties, which increases the excretion of cholic acid and bilirubin. Radix et Rhizoma Rhei *(da huang)* is a very versatile herb. It suppresses Na-K-ATPase, collects water and electrolytes from the colon, stimulates peristalsis and bile secretion, facilitates the coagulation of blood, and has broad-spectrum antibacterial activity. Cornu Antelopis *(ling yang jiao)* is a very strong drug for febrile disorders and is used as a sedative and to control convulsions. Radix Astragali Membranacei *(huang qi),* Radix Codonopsitis Pilosulae *(dang shen),* and Radix Scutellariae Baicalensis *(huang qin)* are uterine inhibitors. Semen Cuscutae Chinensis *(tu si zi)* helps regulate hormone levels during pregnancy. Other herbs such as Herba Lysimachiae *(jin qian cao),* which clear heat and drain dampness, are bacteriostatic but also relieve spasms of the blood vessels and bile ducts. There is evidence that the herbs in this formula may regulate the immune system and stimulate the production of leukocytic interferon. They also inhibit the duplication of HBV (human hepatitis virus) in vitro.

EFFICACY: In a study of 78 cases treated daily with this formula, 76 were cured after one month. In the other two patients, herbal treatment did not work very well and they were thus referred for combined biomedical-traditional Chinese medical treatment.

Hepatic Cholestasis of Pregnancy

This is an uncommon hereditary disorder. Estrogens apparently provoke an insufficiency of hepatic enzymes. This results in an elevated serum conjugated bilirubin level without any other hepatic disorder. Bile salts may deposit into the placenta, however, and may cause fetal distress syndrome. The disease is characterized by gastrointestinal complaints and jaundice. Symptomatic treatment, ion-exchange resin, and administration of bile salts are used to diminish jaundice and relieve itching. Phenothiazines are contraindicated in the treatment of itching because they will intensify the jaundice.

In traditional Chinese medicine this condition corresponds to one type of yang jaundice. Disturbance of the normal metabolic heat and fluids due to pregnancy, combined with dysfunction of the Liver and Spleen, results in bile spilling over from the Gall Bladder to the skin. The more injured the blood and yin, the more heat will manifest with such symptoms as thirst, irritability, itching, and a red tongue.

Herbal treatment

STRATEGY: Clear the heat, eliminate the dampness.

Cornu Bubali *(shui niu jiao)* 30g
Herba Artemisiae Yinchenhao *(yin chen hao)* 15g
Radix Rehmanniae Glutinosae *(sheng di huang)* 12g
Cortex Moutan Radicis *(mu dan pi)* 9g
Radix Paeoniae Rubrae *(chi shao)* 9g
Rhizoma Phragmitis Communis Recens *(xian lu gen)* 9g
Rhizoma Smilacis Glabrae *(tu fu ling)* 9g
Fructus Gardeniae Jasminoidis *(zhi zi)* 9g
Semen Coicis Lachryma-jobi *(yi yi ren)* 12g
Semen Plantaginis *(che qian zi)* 9g
Radix Ledebouriellae Divaricatae *(fang feng)* 3g

METHOD: Take daily as a decoction for seven to fourteen days.

MODIFICATIONS:

1. With severe heat, add:
   Rhizoma Coptidis *(huang lian)* 4.5g
   Fructus Forsythiae Suspensae *(lian qiao)* 4.5g

2. With constipation, add:

Radix et Rhizoma Rhei *(da huang)* 3g

ANALYSIS OF FORMULA: Cornu Bubali *(shui niu jiao)*, Herba Artemisiae Yinchenhao *(yin chen hao)*, Cortex Moutan Radicis *(mu dan pi)*, Radix Paeoniae Rubrae *(chi shao)*, Rhizoma Smilacis Glabrae *(tu fu ling)*, Fructus Forsythiae Suspensae *(lian qiao)*, and Rhizoma Coptidis *(huang lian)* all are used to remove heat. These particular herbs are chosen because they remove heat from the blood and also have some effect in relieving toxicity. Herba Artemisiae Yinchenhao *(yin chen hao)* also has the function of relieving jaundice. Cortex Moutan Radicis *(mu dan pi)* and Fructus Gardeniae Jasminoidis *(zhi zi)* clear heat from the Liver. Radix et Rhizoma Rhei *(da huang)* purges heat and softens dry stools; three grams are enough for this purpose. Radix Rehmanniae Glutinosae *(sheng di huang)* and Rhizoma Phragmitis Communis Recens *(xian lu gen)* clear heat and nourish the yin and body fluids in order to revitalize the Organs. Rhizoma Phragmitis Communis Recens *(xian lu gen)* and Semen Plantaginis *(che qian zi)* clear heat through the urine. The purpose of the whole formula is to clear the heat and dampness lodged in the blood, Liver, and Gall Bladder.

MECHANISM OF ACTION: This formula acts as a choleretic (increasing the flow of bile) and increases blood circulation, especially through the Liver. This has the effect of lowering elevated bilirubin levels back to normal.

EFFICACY: In a study of 34 pregnant patients treated for hepatic cholestasis, 29 obtained symptomatic relief and the return of their bilirubin levels to normal within seven to fourteen days. The efficacy rate was thus 85%.

Acute Pyelonephritis

The urinary tract is especially vulnerable to infection during pregnancy. The altered secretion of sex hormones, combined with the physical pressure of the gravid uterus on the ureters and bladder, cause hypotonia and blockage. This contributes to ureterovesical reflux and stasis. *E. Coli* is the offending organism in the majority of cases. Asymptomatic bacteriuria occurs in 42% of pregnant women, and intercurrent pyelonephritis can be expected in approximately 30% of these patients, whereas urinary tract infection will develop in only one to two percent of pregnant women without prior bacteriuria. High fever, chills, tenderness in the renal area, urinary urgency, and polyuria are the main symptoms. There are higher than average incidences of premature delivery and fetal anomaly. If the condition occurs early in pregnancy, tretracyclines, chloramphenicol, or sulfa drugs may not be used because they are highly teratogenic.

In traditional Chinese medicine, what is defined biomedically as acute pyelonephritis is known as painful urinary dysfunction coupled with lumbar pain. This disorder is attributed to heat and dampness in the Bladder. Besides the symptoms listed above, general pain, nausea, vomiting, poor appetite, thirst, coated red tongue, and a rapid pulse have been recorded. As an acute disorder, this is viewed as a case of excess, even though pregnancy is generally characterized by deficiency.

Herbal treatment

STRATEGY: Clear the heat and dampness from the Lower Burner.

Radix Rehmanniae Glutinosae *(sheng di huang)* 18g
Radix Paeoniae Lactiflorae *(bai shao)* 12g
Radix Scutellariae Baicalensis *(huang qin)* 15g
Herba Taraxaci Mongolici cum Radice *(pu gong ying)* 15g
Herba Lysimachiae *(jin qian cao)* 15g
Herba Polygoni Avicularis *(bian xu)* 15g
Herba Dianthi *(qu mai)* 15g
Rhizoma Dioscoreae Hypoglaucae *(bei xie)* 15g
Sclerotium Poriae Cocos *(fu ling)* 12g
Rhizoma Imperatae Cylindricae *(bai mao gen)* 30g
Tips of Radix Glycyrrhizae Uralensis *(gan cao shao)* 6g

METHOD: Take daily as a decoction for two weeks.

ANALYSIS OF FORMULA: Herba Taraxaci Mongolici cum Radice *(pu gong ying)*, Herba Lysimachiae *(jin qian cao)*, Rhizoma Dioscoreae Hypoglaucae *(bei xie)*, Herba Polygoni Avicularis *(bian xu)*, and Herba Dianthi *(qu mai)* clear heat from the Lower Burner; this is especially true of the latter three herbs, which are often used in treating urinary tract infection. Radix Rehmanniae Glutinosae *(sheng di huang)* and Radix Paeoniae Lactiflorae *(bai shao)* clear heat and replenish the yin of the Kidneys, but their fluid-replenishing properties do not suppress the appetite. Radix Scutellariae Baicalensis *(huang qin)* clears heat and helps prevent miscarriage. Rhizoma Imperatae Cylindricae *(bai mao gen)* clears heat and is helpful when there is hematuria. While Radix Glycyrrhizae Uralensis *(gan cao)* clears heat, its thin tips, known as *gan cao shao,* are especially useful in treating urinary urgency.

MECHANISM OF ACTION: Herba Taraxaci Mongolici cum Radice *(pu gong ying)*, Herba Lysimachiae *(jin qian cao)*, Rhizoma Dioscoreae Hypoglaucae *(bei xie)*, Herba Dianthi *(qu mai)*, and Herba Polygoni Avicularis *(bian xu)* are broad-spectrum bacteriostatics, effective against aerobic and anaerobic microorganisms. Radix Rehmanniae Glutinosae *(sheng di huang)* and Radix Paeoniae Lactiflorae *(bai shao)* lower the pain threshold, bring down fever, and lower blood platelet viscosity. Radix Scutellariae Baicalensis *(huang qin)* is bacteriostatic and relaxes the uterine muscle. Rhizoma Imperatae Cylindricae *(bai mao gen)* shortens the bleeding time and the clotting time, and increases vascular permeability, which increases urinary output. Radix Glycyrrhizae Uralensis *(gan cao)* has a mild cortisone-like action and is a diuretic.

EFFICACY: In one study this formula was used in treating 96 patients with chronic and acute pyelonephritis. Antibiotics were added to the treatment regimen when the fever went above 38°C or septicemia was present, which included all the acute patients. Forty-seven out of 50 acute patients, and 42 out of 46 chronic patients, were cured. No adverse outcome was recorded in any of the pregnancies.

Spontaneous Abortion — Threatened or Recurrent

The main causes of spontaneous abortion are chromosomal defects, acute infection, endocrine disorders, uterine defects, and poisoning. Immune disorders also play an important role (for example, maternal-fetal blood type or rhesus incompatibility). Recurrent spontaneous abortion (RSA) is usually due to recurrent factors rather than accidental causes.

Progestins or hCG are the common hormones used in treatment. Sedatives are sometimes used as well.

In traditional Chinese medicine the Spleen qi and the Kidneys are responsible for the growth of the fetus and for the relaxation of the uterus. Deficiency of the Spleen qi or of the Kidneys may therefore endanger the pregnancy. Excessive heat from the fetus may also disturb a normal pregnancy.

Herbal treatment

Spontaneous Abortion Formula 1

INDICATIONS: Deficiency of the Spleen qi or Kidneys with lower abdominal pain, lower back pain, and vaginal bleeding.

Radix Codonopsitis Pilosulae *(dang shen)* 12g

Rhizoma Atractylodis Macrocephalae *(bai zhu)* 12g

Radix Paeoniae Lactiflorae *(bai shao)* 12g

Radix Scutellariae Baicalensis *(huang qin)* 12g

Semen Cuscutae Chinensis *(tu si zi)* 12g

Radix Dipsaci Asperi *(xu duan)* 12g

Cortex Eucommiae Ulmoidis *(du zhong)* 12g

Ramulus Sangjisheng *(sang ji sheng)* 12g

Ramulus Perillae Frutescentis *(su geng)* 12g

Pedicellus Cucurbitae Moschatae *(nan gua di)* 12g

Radix Boehmeriae *(zhu ma gen)* 12g

ANALYSIS OF FORMULA: Radix Codonopsitis Pilosulae *(dang shen)* and Rhizoma Atractylodis Macrocephalae *(bai zhu)* tonify the qi and thus help the growth of the fetus. Ramulus Perillae Frutescentis *(su geng)* regulates the flow of qi. The latter two herbs, along with Radix Scutellariae Baicalensis *(huang qin)*, are known by modern research to have a relaxing effect on the uterus. Radix Paeoniae Lactiflorae *(bai shao)* relieves pain by relaxing spasms. Radix Dipsaci Asperi *(xu duan)*, Cortex Eucommiae Ulmoidis *(du zhong)*, Ramulus Sangjisheng *(sang ji sheng)*, and Semen Cuscutae Chinensis *(tu si zi)*, through endocrine action, promote the growth of the fetus and of the uterus. Both traditional Chinese medicine and contemporary research concur that it is necessary for the uterus to grow at the same rate as the fetus, otherwise the blood supply will become insufficient. Pedicellus Cucurbitae Moschatae *(nan gua di)* strengthens the Womb and nourishes the fetus. Radix Boehmeriae *(zhu ma gen)* stops vaginal bleeding and prevents miscarriage.

MECHANISM OF ACTION: This formula has been shown to have three functions: to relax the uterus, increase the endocrine output of the corpus luteum, and promote the growth of the uterine muscle and of the fetus.

EFFICACY: This formula has proven effective in preventing 80-90% of cases of threatened abortion.

Spontaneous Abortion Formula 2

INDICATIONS: Excessive heat form the fetus with thirst, constipation, and a red tongue. This is the most common type of RSA.

Herba Artemisiae Yinchenhao *(yin chen hao)* 15g
Fructus Gardeniae Jasminoidis *(zhi zi)*................................. 12g
Cooked Radix et Rhizoma Rhei *(zhi da huang)* 9g
Radix Scutellariae Baicalensis *(huang qin)*............................ 12g
Radix Paeoniae Lactiflorae *(bai shao)* 9g
Radix Glycyrrhizae Uralensis *(gan cao)* 6g
Fructus Citri Aurantii *(zhi ke)*...................................... 6g

Radix Boehmeriae *(zhu ma gen)*..15 g

ANALYSIS OF FORMULA: Herba Artemisiae Yinchenhao *(yin chen hao)*, Fructus Gardeniae Jasminoidis *(zhi zi)*, Radix Scutellariae Baicalensis *(huang qin)*, and Radix et Rhizoma Rhei *(da huang)* all serve to eliminate heat. Cooking *da huang* will reduce its purgative properties. Radix et Rhizoma Rhei *(da huang)* and Radix Glycyrrhizae Uralensis *(gan cao)* clear toxic heat from the fetus.

MECHANISM OF ACTION: This formula acts as an immune regulator and reduces the titer of ABO antibodies.

EFFICACY: In one study, this formula was effective in preventing miscarriage in about 80% of cases due to ABO blood type incompatibility.

Acupuncture treatment

In the author's experience, acupuncture is not indicated for cases of threatened abortion or RSA.

Ectopic Pregnancy

Ninety-five percent of ectopic pregnancies are tubal pregnancies, thus the two terms are often used interchangeably.

In traditional Chinese medicine, ectopic pregnancy, often accompanied by lower abdominal pain and tenderness and uterine bleeding after secondary amenorrhea, is diagnosed as stagnant blood in the Lower Burner. The flow of qi in the Intestines nearly stops and constipation follows. The tongue is sometimes purple.

Herbal treatment

NOTE: Patients must be hospitalized for treatment. Ectopic pregnancies can become life-threatening very quickly. In the past, many hospitals in China did not have access to laparoscopic technology. Depending on the situation, suspected ectopic pregnancies were either treated with surgery or herbal medicine. In present-day China, all larger hospitals do perform laparoscopy for early diagnosis. The standard of care is either micro-surgery or injection of methotrexate to kill the embryo. Thereafter, herbal treatment is given to help in the absorption of any residual blood, maintain the patency of the uterine tubes, or to expel the dead embryo. Patients are discharged when the hCG levels have normalized.

INDICATIONS: For status post surgery or methotrexate injection for ectopic pregnancy.

Radix Salviae Miltiorrhizae *(dan shen)*.....................................15g
Radix Paeoniae Rubrae *(chi shao)* 15g
Semen Persicae *(tao ren)*..9g
Rhizoma Sparganii Stoloniferi *(san leng)*...................................9g
Rhizoma Curcumae Ezhu *(e zhu)*...6g

MODIFICATION:

With constipation and excessive heat, add:

Radix et Rhizoma Rhei *(da huang)*..9g
Mirabilitum *(mang xiao)* 9g
Cortex Magnoliae Officinalis *(hou po)*......................................6g
Fructus Citri seu Ponciri Immaturus *(zhi shi)* 6g

ANALYSIS OF FORMULA: Radix Salviae Miltiorrhizae *(dan shen)*, Radix Paeoniae Rubrae *(chi shao)*, and Semen Persicae *(tao ren)* invigorate the blood and remove blood stasis. Rhizoma Sparganii Stoloniferi *(san leng)* and Rhizoma Curcumae Ezhu *(e zhu)* are used to break up blood stasis and promote the flow of qi in order to alleviate the pain. If needed, Radix et Rhizoma Rhei *(da huang)* can be used as a purgative; it also has the advantage of dispelling blood stasis.

MECHANISM OF ACTION: This formula has been shown to have thrombolytic action, resulting in improved blood flow and hemostasis. Fibrinolytic action was also observed when old blood clots are fibrotic.

These findings are consistent with the traditional Chinese medical concept of bleeding due to blood stasis.

EFFICACY: In one study, treatment was successful in 60-80% of cases. Best results were observed when serum hCG levels were normal. Of 885 successfully cured cases, 75 were cured within 15 days, 279 within 30 days, and 531 within 60 days.[1] "Cured" in this study referred to the absence of vaginal bleeding and pelvic pain, and the disappearance or significant shrinkage of the pelvic mass (ruptured tube, clot, and fibrous tissue). In addition, normal menstruation was restored.

Acupuncture treatment

The use of acupuncture for treating this condition has been mentioned, but no documented evidence suggests its efficacy.

Hyperemesis Gravidarum (Morning Sickness)

Vomiting during pregnancy is considered normal, but if it becomes severe, ketone bodies will appear in the urine and the patient will need to be hospitalized.

In traditional Chinese medicine, morning sickness is considered to be the result of damp stagnation in the Stomach due to fetal qi rising in excess. It is best to give treatment before the symptoms become severe.

Herbal treatment

Besides nausea and vomiting, patients often complain of fatigue and thirst with no desire to drink, and have a greasy tongue coating. The treatment strategy is to resolve the dampness and redirect the flow of qi downward.

Herba Agastaches seu Pogostemi *(huo xiang)* 6g
Ramulus Perillae Frutescentis *(su geng)* 6g
Ginger-prepared Rhizoma Pinelliae Ternatae *(jiang ban xia)* 6g
Pericarpium Arecae Catechu *(da fu pi)* 6g

Terra Flava Usta *(fu long gan)*..12g
Rhizoma Zingiberis Officinalis Recens *(sheng jiang)*......................3g
Fructus Amomi Kravanh *(bai dou kou)* 3g
Pericarpium Citri Reticulatae *(chen pi)*....................................6g
Sclerotium Poriae Cocos *(fu ling)*..9g
Rhizoma Coptidis *(huang lian)* 1.5g
Fructus Evodiae Rutaecarpae *(wu zhu yu)*..............................1.5g

ANALYSIS OF FORMULA: Herba Agastaches seu Pogostemi *(huo xiang)*, ginger-prepared Rhizoma Pinelliae Ternatae *(jiang ban xia)*, Pericarpium Citri Reticulatae *(chen pi)*, Sclerotium Poriae Cocos *(fu ling)*, Fructus Amomi Kravanh *(bai dou kou)*, and Pericarpium Arecae Catechu *(da fu pi)* are used here to resolve dampness, in part by aromatically transforming it, and in part through diuresis. Terra Flava Usta *(fu long gan)* and Ramulus Perillae Frutescentis *(su geng)* serve to redirect the flow of qi downward. Rhizoma Coptidis *(huang lian)* and Fructus Evodiae Rutaecarpae *(wu zhu yu)* together harmonize the Stomach.

EFFICACY: In one study, about 90% of patients showed improvement within two days, and most symptoms had disappeared within ten days. Some patients relapsed as a result of dietary or emotional upset.

Hypertension in Pregnancy

The complex of hypertension, edema, and proteinuria manifesting after the twentieth gestational week is defined as pregnancy-induced hypertension (PIH). If the signs and symptoms are severe and accompanied by headache, the condition is called preeclampsia. If the preeclampsia patient develops coma or convulsions, the term eclampsia is used to describe her condition.

Biomedically, PIH is usually treated with sedatives, spasmolytics (for example, magnesium sulfate) and antihypertensives. Diuretics can be used in mild cases.

In traditional Chinese medicine, edema and eclampsia are attributed to impairment of the Liver and Kidneys. As the growth of the fetus depends mostly on the yin, it is the yin of the Liver and Kidneys that is most likely to be deficient. The initial edema is caused by stagnation of the Liver qi. According to five-phase theory, this results in an impairment of the Spleen function (wood over-controlling or "bullying" earth). As the condition develops, the yin is consumed and the balance between yin and yang is lost. Exuberant yang results in such symptoms as irritability, insomnia, and headache. Liver fire stirs and transforms into internal wind, which is marked by convulsions and coma. Pregnant women who are prone to emotional upset or depression are especially at risk. They often develop qi and blood stagnation, which may progress to heat consuming the yin and then to internal wind.

Herbal treatment

The principle is to eliminate the dampness by tonifying the Spleen, and to nourish the yin of the Liver and Kidneys in order to subdue the yang.

Hypertension in Pregnancy Formula 1

INDICATIONS: For patients with edema, mostly of the legs, and no other signs or symptoms.

Rhizoma Atractylodis Macrocephalae *(bai zhu)* 15g
Sclerotium Poriae Cocos *(fu ling)* 15g
Pericarpium Citri Reticulatae *(chen pi)* 9g
Cortex Mori Albae Radicis *(sang bai pi)* 9g
Pericarpium Arecae Catechu *(da fu pi)* 9g
Cortex Zingiberis Rhizomatis *(jiang pi)* 6g
Radix Aucklandiae Lappae *(mu xiang)* 6g

METHOD: Grind the ingredients into a fine powder, and take 6g twice a day.

ANALYSIS OF FORMULA: Rhizoma Atractylodis Macrocephalae *(bai zhu)*, Sclerotium Poriae Cocos *(fu ling)*, and Cortex Zingiberis Rhizomatis *(jiang pʲ)* dispel water by strengthening the Spleen. Pericarpium Citri Reticulatae *(chen pi)*, Pericarpium Arecae Catechu *(da fu pi)*, and Radix Aucklandiae Lappae *(mu xiang)* all promote the flow of qi to further assist in the resolution of dampness. As the Lungs are responsible for water metabolism, Cortex Mori Albae Radicis *(sang bai pi)*, a cold herb which enters the Lung channel, is used as an auxiliary diuretic.

EFFICACY: In a study of 47 pregnant patients with edema, 46 lost a significant amount of body weight after taking the herbal powder for two weeks. No change was noted in the red blood cell volume.

Hypertension in Pregnancy Formula 2

INDICATIONS: Hypertension with thirst, irritability, a feeling of heat in the chest, flushing. The tongue may be red, and the pulse wiry.

Cornu Antelopis *(ling yang jiao)* 1.5g
Ramulus cum Uncis Uncariae *(gou teng)* 30g
Bombyx Batryticatus *(jiang can)* 20g
Lumbricus *(di long)* 20g
Radix Angelicae Sinensis *(dang gui)* 9g
Radix Ligustici Chuanxiong *(chuan xiong)* 9g
Radix Rehmanniae Glutinosae *(sheng di huang)* 30g
Radix Paeoniae Lactiflorae *(bai shao)* 30g

NOTE: The horn of the common goat, Cornu Naemorhedis *(shan yang jiao)*, can be substituted for Cornu Antelopis *(ling yang jiao)*. This is a more economical and conservation-minded option. The dosage is 30g.

MODIFICATIONS:

1. With proteinuria, add:
   Herba Pyrolae Rotundifoliae *(lu xian cao)* 30g
   Herba Leonuri Heterophylli *(yi mu cao)* 30g
   Semen Coicis Lachryma-jobi *(yi yi ren)* 30g
   Radix Dioscoreae Oppositae *(shan yao)* 15g

2. With edema, add:
Rhizoma Atractylodis Macrocephalae *(bai zhu)*........................15g
Sclerotium Poriae Cocos *(fu ling)*.......................................15g

ANALYSIS OF FORMULA: Cornu Antelopis *(ling yang jiao)*, Ramulus cum Uncis Uncariae *(gou teng)*, Bombyx Batryticatus *(jiang can)*, and Lumbricus *(di long)* all subdue excessive Liver yang and calm internal wind. Radix Rehmanniae Glutinosae *(sheng di huang)* and Radix Paeoniae Lactiflorae *(bai shao)* nourish the yin to help control the yang. Radix Angelicae Sinensis *(dang gui)* and Radix Ligustici Chuanxiong *(chuan xiong)* are used here to invigorate and harmonize the blood, thus helping to resolve the heat from blood stasis.

MECHANISM OF ACTION: The main action of this formula on PIH is to normalize the serum levels of TXB_2, PGI, PGE_2, and $PGF_{2\alpha}$ resulting in a decrease in the spasming of small vessels in the placenta and an improvement in maternal circulation. It also affects the biphasic regulation of blood viscosity.

EFFICACY: In a study of 213 patients with PIH, the symptoms in 86 patients were completely resolved. Of the severe cases, over 72% became mild or moderate. Criteria used were symptoms, hypertension, proteinuria, and edema. Blood viscosity returned to normal levels in 83.5% of those cases.

Maternal-Fetal Blood Type Incompatibility

This is an immune disorder involving the mother's and fetus' respective blood groups, as for example ABO hemolytic disease or Rh hemolytic disease. Hemolysis in the fetus or neonate may cause recurrent miscarriage, fetal death, or stillbirth, or the newborn may exhibit the "yellow baby" syndrome which consists of anemia, jaundice, edema, liver and spleen enlargement, and nerve damage. The titers of serum anti-A (or B) IgG, anti-D IgG, and bilirubin are rather greater than normal. Early diagnosis and treatment by uterine exchange transfusion are up-to-date approaches to this condition. Blue light therapy is given to the newborn as an auxiliary measure.

Maternal-fetal blood type incompatibility falls under the traditional disease rubric of "fetal jaundice." Its cause is thought to be stasis of blood producing heat, the effect of which is to give the fetus its yellow color.

Herbal treatment

STRATEGY: Clear the heat and invigorate the blood in the mother and fetus.

Herba Artemisiae Yinchenhao *(yin chen hao)* 15g
Fructus Gardeniae Jasminoidis *(zhi zi)*. 12g
Cooked Radix et Rhizoma Rhei *(zhi da huang)* 9g
Radix Scutellariae Baicalensis *(huang qin)*. 15g
Rhizoma Atractylodis Macrocephalae *(bai zhu)* 9g
Fructus Citri Aurantii *(zhi ke)*. 6g
Herba Leonuri Heterophylli *(yi mu cao)* 12g
Radix Paeoniae Rubrae *(chi shao)* 12g
Radix Boehmeriae *(zhu ma gen)*. 15g
Radix Glycyrrhizae Uralensis *(gan cao)* 3g

METHOD: Take daily as a decoction until delivery.

ANALYSIS OF FORMULA: Herba Artemisiae Yinchenhao *(yin chen hao)*, Fructus Gardeniae Jasminoidis *(zhi zi)*, Radix Scutellariae Baicalensis *(huang qin)*, and cooked Radix et Rhizoma Rhei *(zhi da huang)* mainly clear heat and resolve dampness. Radix Paeoniae Rubrae *(chi shao)* invigorates the flow of blood and dispels blood stasis. As qi is the commander of blood, herbs that regulate the qi are chosen in order to increase the flow of blood. That is why Rhizoma Atractylodis Macrocephalae *(bai zhu)* and Fructus Citri Aurantii *(zhi ke)* are used in this formula. Radix Glycyrrhizae Uralensis *(gan cao)* is used to harmonize the formula, and also for its heat-clearing properties.

MECHANISM OF ACTION: Herba Artemisiae Yinchenhao *(yin chen hao)* and Fructus Gardeniae Jasminoidis *(zhi zi)* lower serum bilirubin levels.

This formula acts by lowering the titers of serum anti-A (or B) IgG and other related globulins. It also lowers blood viscosity and relaxes the uterine muscle. Herba Leonuri Heterophylli *(yi mu cao)*, Radix Scutellariae Baicalensis *(huang qin)*, Herba Artemisiae Yinchenhao *(yin chen hao)*, Cooked Radix et Rhizoma Rhei *(zhi da huang)*, Fructus Gardeniae Jasminoidis *(zhi zi),* and Radix Paeoniae Rubrae *(chi shao)* significantly reduce serum anti-A, B, and D IgG titers in vitro.

EFFICACY: In one study, 49 of 50 women with ABO incompatibility delivered normal, live babies and there was one fetal death. Nine out of ten women with Rh hemolytic disease had successful deliveries, and there was one fetal death. In 31 cases of neonatal ABO hemolytic disease, all lost their jaundice within two months of treatment using the same formula. When treating the newborn, the dosage is half of that for adults, and the formula is administered by enema.

Breech Presentation

The incidence of breech presentation is about three to four percent. Breech presentation is more likely to cause dystocia than is vertex presentation when both pelvis and fetus are of normal size. The physician should anticipate the following difficulties in delivery: premature membrane rupture, prolapse of the umbilical cord, uterine inertia, difficulty in delivering the head, brachial plexus injury in the newborn, and intracranial damage. External version may be attempted between the thirty-second and thirty-sixth weeks of pregnancy, using careful and gentle maneuvers. Even if the conversion is initially successful, the fetus may spontaneously revert to the breech position.

According to the *Classic of Nourishing Life with Acupuncture and Moxibustion (Zhen jiu zi sheng jing)*, conversion from transverse to breech presentation can be accomplished using moxa at BL-67 *(zhi yin)*. Since 1990, laser radiation has been used in China with results similar to those obtained with moxibustion.

Acupuncture treatment

BL-67 *(zhi yin)* bilaterally

MOXIBUSTION: Warm the points 15 minutes daily for five days, or until conversion has occurred.

LASER THERAPY: Use 2 to 3mW HeNe (632.8 nm) laser. Before each treatment check the fetal position by hand palpation. Apply daily for five minutes. Seven treatments constitute a course. Suspend treatment when conversion has occurred. Follow up weekly and repeat treatment if the fetus has reverted to the breech position.

MECHANISM OF ACTION: After moxa or laser stimulation at BL-67 *(zhi yin)*, the frequency of fetal movement is increased and the mother's uterine muscles contract slightly. The exact mechanism responsible for the conversion has yet to be completely explored.

EFFICACY: In a controlled study involving 615 pregnant women with breech presentation of the fetus, those treated obtained conversion in 85% of cases compared with 65.7% spontaneous conversion in the control group. In both groups the umbilical cord was entangled in about 6% of cases.

Herbal treatment

STRATEGY: Tonify the qi and blood, and promote the flow of qi and blood, in order to ameliorate the fetal environment.

Radix Angelicae Sinensis *(dang gui)* 9g
Radix Ligustici Chuanxiong *(chuan xiong)* 9g
Radix Astragali Membranacei *(huang qi)* 9g
Radix Codonopsitis Pilosulae *(dang shen)* 9g
Rhizoma Atractylodis Macrocephalae *(bai zhu)* 9g
Radix Paeoniae Lactiflorae *(bai shao)* 9g

Radix Dipsaci Asperi *(xu duan)*..9g

Fructus Citri Aurantii *(zhi ke)*...9g

Radix Rehmanniae Glutinosae Conquitae *(shu di huang)* 9g

Radix Glycyrrhizae Uralensis *(gan cao)* 9g

METHOD: Take daily as a decoction until conversion occurs.

ANALYSIS OF FORMULA: Radix Astragali Membranacei *(huang qi)*, Radix Codonopsitis Pilosulae *(dang shen)*, Rhizoma Atractylodis Macrocephalae *(bai zhu)*, and Radix Glycyrrhizae Uralensis *(gan cao)* replenish the qi of the mother and fetus. Radix Angelicae Sinensis *(dang gui)*, Radix Ligustici Chuanxiong *(chuan xiong)*, Radix Rehmanniae Glutinosae Conquitae *(shu di huang)*, and Radix Paeoniae Lactiflorae *(bai shao)* tonify the blood of the mother and fetus. Fructus Citri Aurantii *(zhi ke)* regulates the flow of qi in order to benefit the Womb. Radix Dipsaci Asperi *(xu duan)* strengthens the Liver and Kidneys, and invigorates the blood.

EFFICACY: One may expect 80-90% efficacy, but this figure is not supported by controlled studies.

Hydramnios (Excess Amniotic Fluid)

The diagnosis of hydramnios is called for when the volume of amniotic fluid in the third trimester exceeds 2000ml. This condition may be acute or it may develop progressively. The etiology is unknown. Approximately 25% of all cases of hydramnios are associated with fetal abnormality, while the rest are associated with multiple pregnancy, diabetes, or other factors. Hydramnios may accompany hypertension, malposition of the fetus, premature labor, heavy bleeding, and abruptio placentae. Conventional treatment is to induce labor.

From a traditional perspective, hydramnios is due to deficiency of the Kidney and Spleen yang, leading to accumulation of fluid within the Womb. It is not clear why the yang deficiency results in such accumulation, rather than edema in the mother's tissues.

Herbal treatment

STRATEGY: Tonify the Kidneys and Spleen to expel water and protect the fetus.

Cortex Poriae Cocos *(fu ling pi)* 15g
Epicarpium Benincasae Hispidae *(dong gua pi)* 15g
Pericarpium Arecae Catechu *(da fu pi)* 15g
Radix Dioscoreae Oppositae *(shan yao)* 15g
Fructus Nelumbinis Nuciferae *(shi lian zi)* 9g
Semen Dolichoris Lablab *(bian dou)* 15g
Semen Plantaginis *(che qian zi)* 9g
Semen Trigonellae Foeni-graeci *(hu lu ba)* 15g
Radix Dipsaci Asperi *(xu duan)* 9g
Caulis Aristolochiae *(tian xian teng)* 9g
Radix Aristolochiae Fangchi *(fang ji)* 6g

METHOD: Take daily as a decoction for six to ten days until the amount of amniotic fluid visible by ultrasound decreases and the symptoms improve. Follow up with the following maintenance formula:

Sclerotium Poriae Cocos *(fu ling)* 12g
Rhizoma Atractylodis Macrocephalae *(bai zhu)* 6g
Fructus Nelumbinis Nuciferae *(shi lian zi)* 9g
Semen Plantaginis *(che qian zi)* 9g
Radix Dioscoreae Oppositae *(shan yao)* 15g
Pericarpium Arecae Catechu *(da fu pi)* 15g
Semen Trigonellae Foeni-graeci *(hu lu ba)* 9g
Ramulus Sangjisheng *(sang ji sheng)* 9g
Radix Dipsaci Asperi *(xu duan)* 9g
Epicarpium Benincasae Hispidae *(dong gua pi)* 15g
Semen Abutili seu Malvae *(dong kui zi)* 6g
Caulis Aristolochiae *(tian xian teng)* 9g

METHOD: Take daily as a decoction until the volume of amniotic fluid has been reduced significantly, as evidenced by ultrasonography, then take the same formula every other day until delivery.

ANALYSIS OF FORMULA: Ramulus Sangjisheng *(sang ji sheng)*, Radix Dipsaci Asperi *(xu duan)*, Radix Dioscoreae Oppositae *(shan yao)*, and Fructus Nelumbinis Nuciferae *(shi lian zi)* tonify the Kidneys and help resolve the retention of water. Semen Dolichoris Lablab *(bian dou)* and Rhizoma Atractylodis Macrocephalae *(bai zhu)* tonify the Spleen to reinforce its water-transforming function. Cortex Poriae Cocos *(fu ling pi)*, Epicarpium Benincasae Hispidae *(dong gua pi)*, Pericarpium Arecae Catechu *(da fu pi)*, Semen Plantaginis *(che qian zi)*, Semen Trigonellae Foeni-graeci *(hu lu ba)*, Caulis Aristolochiae *(tian xian teng)*, Radix Aristolochiae Fangchi *(fang ji)*, and Semen Abutili seu Malvae *(dong kui zi)* are diurectics useful in cases of severe edema and fluid-filled cavities. Although the mechanism of action has not been studied, patients treated with this formula produce more urine and their amniotic fluid volume decreases.

EFFICACY: In a study of 60 women with hydramnios, 44 of the 46 cases with normal fetuses saw their amniotic fluid volume become normal and gave birth to normal babies. Four women with mildly abnormal fetuses also saw their amniotic fluid level return to normal. Of the ten women with severe fetal abnormality, none showed any reduction in fluid volume. Conversely, the two mothers who had normal fetuses but who did not see their amniotic fluid volume reduced gave birth to normal babies. On average, treatment required ingestion of 12 to 18 decoctions.

Inducing Labor with Acupuncture

According to the traditional Chinese medical literature, the use of acupoints LI-4 *(he gu)* and SP-6 *(san yin jiao)* is forbidden during pregnancy. Since 1970, however, these points have been used to induce labor. Prolonged pregnancy and premature rupture of the membrane are indications for the procedure. A comparative study showed a success rate of 72% for acupuncture (experimental group of 771) versus 70% for oxytocin (comparison group of 118).[2]

INDICATIONS: Prolonged labor, early membrane rupture.

LI-4 *(he gu)*
SP-6 *(san yin jiao)*

METHOD: Needles are inserted ipsilaterally on one side so as to leave one hand and one leg free, and to avoid crossing the heart. Electrical stimulation is applied continuously for six to eight hours at about three Hertz, and at a mild and comfortable intensity. This procedure should be carried out for three consecutive days, with a different side stimulated each day.

MECHANISM OF ACTION: Six different factors have been studied: the type of stimulator, wave form, parity, whether the membrane was stripped or intact, and Bishop pelvic score. It has been found that a ruptured membrane and a Bishop score over seven were the two factors which significantly improved the results, while other factors had no effect. After acupuncture the cervix is softened and dilates more easily, and women experience less pain during labor than with oxytocin. Recent studies show that the ratio of estrogen to progesterone (E_2/P) and the level of $PG_{2\alpha}$ become elevated after acupuncture, while not in normal labor. The serum oxytocin level after acupuncture is not as elevated as in normal or oxytocin-induced labor.

EFFICACY: Another study showed an efficacy rate of 62% for acupuncture (164 cases) as opposed to 70% for artificial membrane rupture plus pitocin drip (53 cases). In the acupuncture group, the success rate was 42% when the membrane was not ruptured, and 80% with a ruptured membrane ($p < 0.05$). When the Bishop score was five or less, the success rate was 45%; this increased to 73% when the Bishop score was six or more ($p < 0.05$). No variations were evidenced with different parities.

Endnotes

1. Another treatment used in China is the intramuscular injection of 2.4mg trichosantin, which is a purified extract of Radix Trichosanthis

Kirilowii *(tian hua fen)*. A skin allergy test should be done two hours beforehand. Patients should stay in bed for 48 hours, and vital signs should be recorded every six hours. For prevention of side effects, 5mg of dexamethasone may be administered intramuscularly twice a day for two days. If hCG levels remain high, treatment may be repeated one week later. Trichosantin can drive trophoblasts to necrosis and eliminate intervillious spaces with fibrosis. In one study of 61 ectopic pregnancies with elevated hCG levels, 35 saw their levels return to normal. In 19 cases the level returned to normal in eight to 14 days, in 15 to 21 days in three cases, and in 22 to 28 days in another two cases. In only two cases did it take more than 28 days for the hCG levels to return to normal. This treatment is often combined with the herbal treatment noted here.

2. These numbers are skewed as the comparison group did not begin to be assembled until 500 cases had been treated with the protocol.

8

Postpartum Complications

Postpartum Heat Stroke

AFTER LABOR THE general state of the mother's health is one of physical fatigue. During the postpartum period, if the environment is so stifling, hot, and humid that the mother cannot dissipate the heat resulting from labor, heat stroke may result. Early symptoms are high fever, heavy perspiration, fatigue, thirst, dizziness, palpitations, and a sensation of fullness in the chest. Later, as a result of electrolyte imbalance and neurological disturbances, more severe signs and symptoms may appear such as flushed face, headache, nausea, vomiting, dry skin, and hypotension. In severe cases fever may reach 40°C (104°F) and coma, delirium, or convulsions may be seen. Withdrawal from the hot and humid environment and symptomatic treatment are important measures. In order to restore homeostasis, bringing the fever down and restoring the water and electrolyte balance are essential.

Traditional Chinese medicine views postpartum heat stroke as a combined pattern of excess and deficiency. Loss of blood during childbirth leads to deficiency of blood and yin; no longer restrained, the yang floats upward to the upper part of the body. External heat (a yang factor) and dampness (a yin factor) invade and cover the Upper Burner and also exhaust the qi. The patient thereupon complains of a sensation of internal heat, sweating on the head but not on the remainder of the body, thirst, palpitations, and insomnia. In severe cases, excessive heat in the Upper Burner may cause coma, convulsions, and delirium.

Herbal treatment

Postpartum Heat Stroke Formula 1

STRATEGY: Reinforce the qi and blood and replenish the yin to check the floating yang.

Radix Pseudostellariae Heterophyllae *(tai zi shen)* 15g
Tuber Ophiopogonis Japonici *(mai men dong)* 9g
Fructus Schisandrae Chinensis *(wu wei zi)* 9g
Radix Astragali Membranacei *(huang qi)* 15g
Radix Glycyrrhizae Uralensis *(gan cao)* 9g
Cortex Cinnamomi Cassiae *(rou gui)* 1.5g
Dry-fried Radix Paeoniae Lactiflorae *(chao bai shao)* 15g

METHOD: Take daily as a decoction. Seven days constitute one course. There should be significant improvement within six hours of taking the formula, but for best results, it should continue to be taken for one week.

MODIFICATIONS:

1. With dripping lochia, add:
   Radix Rubiae Cordifoliae *(qian cao gen)* 15g

2. With insomnia, add:
   Semen Biotae Orientalis *(bai zi ren)* 9g
   Semen Zizyphi Spinosae *(suan zao ren)* 9g

3. With palpitations, add:
   Calcined Os Draconis *(duan long gu)* 15g

4. With constipation, add:
   Fructus Trichosanthis *(gua lou)* 15g

5. With poor appetite and a greasy tongue coating, add:
   Dry-fried Rhizoma Atractylodis Macrocephalae *(chao bai zhu)* 9g

6. With anemia, add:
   Rhizoma Polygonati *(huang jing)* 15g
   Radix Angelicae Sinensis *(dang gui)* 9g

ANALYSIS OF FORMULA: Radix Astragali Membranacei *(huang qi)*, Radix Pseudostellariae Heterophyllae *(tai zi shen)*, and Radix Glycyrrhizae Uralensis *(gan cao)* replenish the qi. Radix Astragali Membranacei *(huang qi)* is also useful for anemia, especially when combined with Radix Angelicae Sinensis *(dang gui)*. Radix Pseudostellariae Heterophyllae *(tai zi shen)* helps the digestion when it is combined with dry-fried Rhizoma Atractylodis Macrocephalae *(chao bai zhu)*. Tuber Ophiopogonis Japonici *(mai men dong)*, Fructus Schisandrae Chinensis *(wu wei zi)*, and dry-fried Radix Paeoniae Lactiflorae *(chao bai shao)* replenish the yin, mostly of the Heart, and check perspiration; according to traditional Chinese medicine, sweat is the fluid of the Heart. Cortex Cinnamomi Cassiae *(rou gui)* is added to mitigate the action of the other substances that tonify the yin, namely Tuber Ophiopogonis Japonici *(mai men dong)* and Radix Paeoniae Lactiflorae *(bai shao)*. Cortex Cinnamomi Cassiae *(rou gui)* is also said to facilitate the transformation of yin into yang. Radix Rubiae Cordifoliae *(qian cao gen)* invigorates the blood and checks bleeding due to blood stasis. Semen Biotae Orientalis *(bai zi ren)* and Semen Zizyphi Spinosae *(suan zao ren)* are sedatives useful in treating yin deficiency. Calcined Os Draconis *(duan long gu)* nourishes the Heart, soothes the nerves, and holds the exuberant yang and perspiration in check. Fructus Trichosanthis *(gua lou)* very gently moistens the Intestines and alleviates constipation. Rhizoma Atractylodis Macrocephalae *(bai zhu)* replenishes the Spleen and Stomach. In its dry-fried form, it is less tonifying but is more effective in transforming dampness and draining it through the urine.

MECHANISM OF ACTION: The mechanism of action of this formula has not been explained.

EFFICACY: In one study of 90 puerperal women with heat stroke treated with this formula, 62 were completely relieved of symptoms after one or two courses of treatment, while 24 showed good improvement. The remaining four saw no improvement within several hours, at which time biomedical pharmaceuticals were added to their treatment.

Postpartum Heat Stroke Formula 2

STRATEGY: Harmonize the yin and yang, and dispel pathogens through sweating.

Radix Bupleuri *(chai hu)*..6g
Wine-fried Radix Scutellariae Baicalensis *(jiu huang qin)*................6g
Rhizoma Pinelliae Ternatae *(ban xia)* 9g
Caulis Bambusae in Taeniis *(zhu ru)* 4.5g
Radix Codonopsitis Pilosulae *(dang shen)* 6g
Radix Angelicae Sinensis *(dang gui)*.......................................9g
Dry-fried Radix Paeoniae Lactiflorae *(chao bai shao)*.....................9g
Fructus Citri Aurantii *(zhi ke)*...4.5g
Radix Glycyrrhizae Uralensis *(gan cao)* 3g

METHOD: Take as a decoction for two days.

ANALYSIS OF FORMULA: This is the classical formula Minor Bupleurum Decoction *(xiao chai hu tang)* from the *Discussion of Cold-induced Disorders (Shang han lun)*, as modified by Dr. Ha Li-Tian, a famous traditional Chinese gynecologist who was active in Tianjin from the 1960s through the 1980s. Radix Angelicae Sinensis *(dang gui)* and Radix Paeoniae Lactiflorae *(bai shao)* replenish the yin and blood. Radix Paeoniae Lactiflorae *(bai shao)* is easier to digest and less heavy when dry-fried. Radix Codonopsitis Pilosulae *(dang shen)* and Radix Glycyrrhizae Uralensis *(gan cao)* replenish the qi in order to promote the harmony of yin and yang. Radix Bupleuri *(chai hu)* and Radix Scutellariae Baicalensis *(huang qin)* clear the heat that is half interior and half exterior. Radix Scutellariae Baicalensis *(huang qin)* is more effective in the Upper Burner

124

when it is cooked with rice wine. Fructus Citri Aurantii *(zhi ke)*, Rhizoma Pinelliae Ternatae *(ban xia),* and Caulis Bambusae in Taeniis *(zhu ru)* resolve phlegm-dampness and soothe the Stomach.

MECHANISM OF ACTION: This formula strengthens the body resistance, dispels external pathogens, and restores the normal relationship between the body and the external environment. Its approach is different from that of the first formula, which emphasizes tonification. While its pharmacological mechanism has yet to be explained, and there is no scientific evidence regarding its efficacy, Dr. Ha Li-Tian has described patients being cured within two days using this formula.

Puerperal and Postoperative Urinary Retention

Urinary retention is defined as a condition when the patient fails to void even though the contents of her bladder exceed 500ml. After delivery or gynecologic surgery, pain resulting from strain on the voluntary muscles involved in urination may cause retention. A bruised or edematous bladder after a difficult delivery, pain due to episiotomy, vaginal plastic procedures, the placement of sutures near the urethra, or urethral edema can make voiding difficult or impossible. Continuous drainage (urethral drainage, sometimes suprapubic) probably poses fewer problems than frequent intermittent catheterizations.

In traditional Chinese medicine, the Bladder connects with the Kidneys and is also related to the activities of the Triple Burner in general and the Lower Burner in particular. Kidney yang deficiency and dysfunction of the Triple Burner may result in urinary retention or dribbling urination.

Herbal treatment

Urinary Retention Formula 1

Ramulus Cinnamomi Cassiae *(gui zhi)* 9g
Baked Rhizoma Atractylodis Macrocephalae *(wei bai zhu)* 9g

Sclerotium Polypori Umbellati *(zhu ling)* 12g
Sclerotium Poriae Cocos *(fu ling)* 15g
Rhizoma Alismatis Orientalis *(ze xie)* 15g
Radix Paeoniae Lactiflorae *(bai shao)* 21g
Cortex Phellodendri *(huang bai)* 9g
Rhizoma Acori Graminei *(shi chang pu)* 3g
Rhizoma Atractylodis *(cang zhu)* 9g
Honey-toasted Radix Glycyrrhizae Uralensis *(zhi gan cao)* 6g

METHOD: Take the decoction for one or two days.

MODIFICATIONS:

1. With intolerance to cold, add:
   Radix Lateralis Aconiti Carmichaeli Praeparata *(fu zi)* 6g

2. With fatigue, add:
   Radix Codonopsitis Pilosulae *(dang shen)* 15g
   Radix Astragali Membranacei *(huang qi)* 15g

3. With fullness of the abdomen, add:
   Radix Linderae Strychnifoliae *(wu yao)* 9g
   Fructus Foeniculi Vulgaris *(xiao hui xiang)* 9g

4. With dark urine, add:
   Herba Taraxaci Mongolici cum Radice *(pu gong ying)* 30g
   Rhizoma Imperatae Cylindricae *(bai mao gen)* 30g

ANALYSIS OF FORMULA: Ramulus Cinnamomi Cassiae *(gui zhi)*, a warm, acrid herb, promotes the flow of qi and blood, and promotes sweating and voiding. When combined with Rhizoma Atractylodis Macrocephalae *(bai zhu)* and Sclerotium Poriae Cocos *(fu ling)*, it improves the function of the Lower Burner and benefits the Bladder. Sclerotium Polypori Umbellati *(zhu ling)*, Rhizoma Alismatis Orientalis *(ze xie)*, Sclerotium Poriae Cocos *(fu ling)*, and Rhizoma Atractylodis *(cang zhu)* are diuretics. Rhizoma Acori Graminei *(shi chang pu)* removes dampness from the Triple Burner. Radix Paeoniae Lactiflorae *(bai shao)* replenishes the Kidney yin and also relieves pain and strengthens the Bladder. Tips of Radix Glycyrrhizae Uralensis *(gan cao shao)* and Cortex Phellodendri *(huang bai)* clear heat

126

from the Bladder. Radix Lateralis Aconiti Carmichaeli Praeparata *(fu zi)* reinforces the actions of Radix Codonopsitis Pilosulae *(dang shen)*, Radix Astragali Membranacei *(huang qi)*, and Ramulus Cinnamomi Cassiae *(gui zhi)* in increasing the qi and its flow. Radix Linderae Strychnifoliae *(wu yao)* and Fructus Foeniculi Vulgaris *(xiao hui xiang)* regulate the flow of qi in the Lower Burner. Herba Taraxaci Mongolici cum Radice *(pu gong ying)* and Rhizoma Imperatae Cylindricae *(bai mao gen)*, in combination with Cortex Phellodendri *(huang bai)*, clear heat from the Bladder.

MECHANISM OF ACTION: The pharmacological mechanism of action in this formula has yet to be studied.

EFFICACY: In one study, after 20 patients with postpartum urinary retention were treated for one to two days using this formula, all of them voided normally.

Urinary Retention Formula 2

STRATEGY: Clear heat, drain dampness, and promote normal urination.

Herba Polygoni Avicularis *(bian xu)* 9g
Herba Dianthi *(qu mai)* 9g
Caulis Mutong *(mu tong)* 6g
Semen Plantaginis *(che qian zi)* 9g
Talcum *(hua shi)* 12g
Fructus Gardeniae Jasminoidis *(zhi zi)* 6g
Tips of Radix Glycyrrhizae Uralensis *(gan cao shao)* 3g
Cortex Phellodendri *(huang bai)* 9g

METHOD: Take as a decoction for one or two days.

MODIFICATIONS:

1. With fatigue, add:
   Radix Astragali Membranacei *(huang qi)* 15g
   Radix Codonopsitis Pilosulae *(dang shen)* 15g

2. With constipation, add:

   Mirabilitum *(mang xiao)*..9g

3. With insomnia, add:

   Succinum *(hu po)*..3g

ANALYSIS OF FORMULA: Herba Polygoni Avicularis *(bian xu)*, Herba Dianthi *(qu mai)*, Caulis Mutong *(mu tong)*, Semen Plantaginis *(che qian zi)*, Talcum *(hua shi)*, Fructus Gardeniae Jasminoidis *(zhi zi)*, and Cortex Phellodendri *(huang bai)* clear heat and drain dampness from the Lower Burner. The tips of Radix Glycyrrhizae Uralensis *(gan cao shao)* are especially useful for urinary urgency. Radix Astragali Membranacei *(huang qi)* and Radix Codonopsitis Pilosulae *(dang shen)* tonify the qi; this helps regulate the Triple Burner, especially the Lower Burner, which is responsible for urination. Succinum *(hu po)* is a sedative, but is also a useful diuretic and hemostatic in acute urinary infection.

Acupuncture treatment

Body acupuncture

CV-3 *(zhong ji):* if there is a scar at this point, use ST-29 *(gui lai)* on the available side instead

SP-6 *(san yin jiao)*

SP-9 *(yin ling quan)*

METHOD: The needle at CV-3 *(zhong ji)* is inserted deeply into the abdominal fascia. The sensation should extend to the area of the vulva. Use mild to moderate stimulation, 30 minutes daily, for one to three days.

MODIFICATIONS:

1. With fatigue, add:

   ST-36 *(zu san li)*

2. With intolerance to cold, add:

   BL-23 *(shen shu)* or BL-28 *(pang guang shu)*, using moxibustion

ANALYSIS OF POINT COMBINATION: CV-3 *(zhong ji)*, ST-29 *(gui lai)*, and SP-9 *(yin ling quan)* control urination. SP-6 *(san yin jiao)* is essential for all kinds of obstetrical and gynecological disorders owing to its regulatory effect on the Kidney, Liver, and Spleen channels.

MECHANISM OF ACTION: Acupuncture normalizes the function of the Bladder whether it is hypertonic or hypotonic. During acupuncture, parasympathetic nerves are stimulated via the pelvic afferent fibers. Urination centers are located in the spinal cord, midbrain, and pons. In the midbrain, the bladder contraction center is located in the lateral reticular part of the para aquatuo greg (PAG). The bladder relaxation center is located in the medial reticular part of the PAG. In an experiment with rabbits, both parts were found to overlap, and both centers are affected by needling point BL-32 *(ci liao)*. In clinical practice, CV-3 *(zhong ji)*, SP-6 *(san yin jiao)*, and SP-9 *(yin ling quan)* are equivalent. In another experiment involving rabbits, an electrode implanted into the PAG area was used to suppress normal bladder contraction. Needling point BL-32 *(ci liao)* reversed the inhibition.

EFFICACY: In one study, 78 out of 80 women with puerperal or postoperative urinary retention obtained relief after three days of acupuncture treatment. When necessary, catheterization with periodic clamping was used during treatment. Another study showed that of 40 women treated with acupuncture, 15 were cured after one treatment, and 13 more after a second treatment. Ten women required ten days of treatment before experiencing relief, and two had no results.

Ear acupuncture

Ureter or Bladder
Kidney or Urethra
Triple Burner or Sympathetic

METHOD: Select three or four points. Locate the precise point by finding the spot that is most sensitive to pressure in the area of the point. Tiny magnetic balls ("BBs") are secured on one ear with adhesive tape. They should be pressed forcefully for two minutes each, five times daily. After four days repeat the procedure on the other ear, leaving the balls in place for four days if urination remains abnormal.

If the patient has a greasy tongue coating or poor appetite, use the Triple Burner point. If she is nervous, select the Sympathetic point.

MECHANISM OF ACTION: All of the points above have a reflex action on the urinary tract, possibly via the urination center in the brain stem.

Insufficient Lactation

Milk is produced and moved from the acini towards the nipple by the contractile myoepithelial cells. These are stimulated by oxytocin released by the posterior pituitary in response to the infant's nursing. The average volume of milk produced daily after the third postpartum day is around 240-300cc. Occasionally the paucity of mammary glands reduces the amount of milk produced, but the usual cause of insufficient lactation is inhibition due to such problems as stress, puerperal hemorrhage, infection, or diarrhea. Breast engorgement or edema of the areola can also cause the infant to nurse poorly in spite of an adequate milk production. The conventional treatment is usually symptomatic.

Traditional Chinese medicine views blood as the material basis for milk. Lactation is related to the health of the yang brightness channel. The yang brightness channel contains much of both qi and blood: proper downward movement is required for normal menstruation, and proper upward movement for normal lactation. This idea is clearly stated in *Corrected Fine Formulas for Women (Jiao zhen fu ren liang fang)* by the sixteenth-century author Xue Li-Zhai: "Blood is the essence of water and grains and regulates the Organs. In men it is transformed into sperm, while in women it ascends to become milk and descends to become menstrual fluid." Insufficient lactation is thus classified as either qi and blood deficiency, or as a condition of excess resulting from qi and blood stagnation. Differentiation is based largely on whether the breasts are tender,

which indicates excess, and on other general systemic signs and symptoms. Fever, local redness and swelling, and tender, enlarged lymph nodes
in the axilla are other signs of excess.

Women are especially vulnerable to external pathogenic factors during
the postpartum period. A combination of wind and dampness is typically
responsible for blocking the flow of qi to the breasts. It is also possible for
conditions of deficiency and excess to coexist.

Herbal treatment

Insufficient Lactation Formula 1

STRATEGY: Replenish the qi and blood in order to promote lactation.

Radix Astragali Membranacei *(huang qi)* 12g
Radix Codonopsitis Pilosulae *(dang shen)* 12g
Radix Angelicae Sinensis *(dang gui)* 12g
Radix Trichosanthis Kirilowii *(tian hua fen)* 12g
Tuber Ophiopogonis Japonici *(mai men dong)* 9g
Rhizoma Atractylodis Macrocephalae *(bai zhu)* 9g
Semen Vaccariae Segetalis *(wang bu liu xing)* 12g
Squama Manitis Pentadactylae *(chuan shan jia)* 6g
Medulla Tetrapanacis Papyriferi *(tong cao)* 3g

METHOD: Take daily as a decoction, for five days, along with two pig's feet.
The pig's feet may be cooked separately or with the decoction. It is best if
the pig's feet are cooked without salt.

ANALYSIS OF FORMULA: Radix Astragali Membranacei *(huang qi)*, Radix
Codonopsitis Pilosulae *(dang shen)*, and Rhizoma Atractylodis Macrocephalae *(bai zhu)* replenish the qi and strengthen the Spleen. Radix
Angelicae Sinensis *(dang gui)*, Radix Trichosanthis Kirilowii *(tian hua
fen)*, and Tuber Ophiopogonis Japonici *(mai men dong)* nourish the blood
and vital essence. Pig's feet are a traditional remedy used by the Chinese to
tonify the blood and promote lactation. Semen Vaccariae Segetalis *(wang*

bu liu xing) and Squama Manitis Pentadactylae *(chuan shan jia)* assist in promoting lactation. Medulla Tetrapanacis Papyriferi *(tong cao)* guides the functions of the other herbs toward the same goal.

MECHANISM OF ACTION: The mechanism of action has yet to be explained.

EFFICACY: In one study, the efficacy of this formula was 95%, with one-third of patients showing significant improvement within one to six days.

Insufficient Lactation Formula 2

INDICATIONS: Scanty lactation with puerperal fever caused by exogenous pathogenic factors.

STRATEGY: Dispel external wind, nourish the blood, and eliminate stasis in order to promote lactation.

Radix Ledebouriellae Divaricatae *(fang feng)* 4.5g
Cortex Erythrinae *(hai tong pi)* 12g
Herba Siegesbeckiae *(xi xian cao)* 9g
Radix Clematidis *(wei ling xian)* 9g
Radix Dipsaci Asperi *(xu duan)* 12g
Radix Angelicae Sinensis *(dang gui)* 12g
Radix Paeoniae Lactiflorae *(bai shao)* 9g
Radix Cynanchi Baiwei *(bai wei)* 9g
Herba Artemisiae Anomalae *(liu ji nu)* 12g
Semen Vaccariae Segetalis *(wang bu liu xing)* 6g
Squama Manitis Pentadactylae *(chuan shan jia)* 4.5g
Pericarpium Citri Reticulatae Viride *(qing pi)* 4.5g
Herba cum Radice Asari *(xi xin)* 1.5g

METHOD: Take daily as a decoction.

ANALYSIS OF FORMULA: Radix Ledebouriellae Divaricatae *(fang feng)*,

Cortex Erythrinae *(hai tong pi)*, Radix Clematidis *(wei ling xian)*, Herba Siegesbeckiae *(xi xian cao)*, Radix Cynanchi Baiwei *(bai wei)*, and Herba cum Radice Asari *(xi xin)* dispel external wind and dampness. Radix Dipsaci Asperi *(xu duan)*, Radix Angelicae Sinensis *(dang gui)*, and Radix Paeoniae Lactiflorae *(bai shao)* replenish the Kidneys and nourish the blood. Herba Artemisiae Anomalae *(liu ji nu)*, Pericarpium Citri Reticulatae Viride *(qing pi)*, Semen Vaccariae Segetalis *(wang bu liu xing)*, and Squama Manitis Pentadactylae *(chuan shan jia)* promote the flow of qi and blood.

Acupuncture treatment

SI-1 *(shao ze)*
CV-17 *(shan zhong)*
ST-18 *(ru gen)*

METHOD: The needles should be retained for 20 minutes daily until results are achieved.

MODIFICATION: With blood deficiency, add BL-17 *(ge shu)*.

EXPLANATION OF POINTS: CV-17 *(shan zhong)*, the influential point of the qi, enhances the flow of qi throughout the body and thereby influences lactation. The Stomach channel is rich with qi and blood; ST-18 *(ru gen)* is located just below the breast on this channel. Stimulating this point can promote the flow of qi and blood in the breast. The Small Intestine channel is paired with the Heart channel. Since the Heart governs the blood, needling SI-1 *(shao ze)* will help regulate the flow of qi and blood, thereby freeing the production of milk. If there is blood deficiency, BL-17 *(ge shu)*, the influential point of blood, is also used.

MECHANISM OF ACTION: The mother's prolactin level elevates significantly after acupuncture. In an experiment involving rats, blood prolactin levels were higher after needling CV-17 *(shan zhong)* than after needling ST-36 *(zu san li)*. This reflects the importance of the specificity of acupuncture points when used to stimulate lactation. If the melatonin-secreting region or the norepinephrinic fibers are destroyed in the rat brain, no elevation of the prolactin level will be found. These experiments suggest that acupuncture on these special points induces lactation via a neuroendocrine pathway.

Puerperal Morbidity

Febrile morbidity in the puerperium is defined as a temperature elevation to 38°C (100.4°C) or more occurring after the first 24 hours postpartum, on two or more occasions within six hours of each other. The most frequent causes are genital or urinary tract infection and breast problems. The most common pathogens include anaerobic, non-hemolytic streptococci, coliform bacteria and others. Mycoplasmas and viruses have been detected in higher concentrations in the genital tract and may be the cause of chronic febrile conditions.

A low-grade fever in the second or third day postpartum is often caused by retention of lochia or by a saprophytic infection of retained fragments of fetal membranes. The majority of patients with puerperal fever present with endometritis, urinary infection, or mastitis. (These topics are considered in other chapters.) Other possible medical complications such as appendicitis, pneumonia, or enterogastritis should also be kept in mind. Diagnosis must be clear and based on history, physical examination, and laboratory studies. Antibiotics, fluid balance, and symptomatic treatment are commonly suggested in biomedicine.

Traditional Chinese medicine regards puerperal fever mainly as an attack by external pathogens when the qi and blood are suddenly lost after delivery. Some blood remains in the Womb; this causes local blood stasis, which produces heat. The exhausted channels are vulnerable to exogenous pathogenic factors, with the resulting symptoms of fever, chills, and signs of dampness and heat.

TREATMENT STRATEGY: For puerperal fever caused by pelvic infection, see Chapter 4. Herba Leonuri Heterophylli *(yi mu cao)* is usually added to those herbal treatments in order to direct the action of the other herbs to the genital tract, and to induce uterine contractions. The formula below is suitable for puerperal fever including mild or moderate genital tract infections, breast engorgement, or influenza, as long as the presentation is consistent with the formula's traditional functions.

Puerperal Morbidity Formula 1

STRATEGY: Replenish the qi and blood, and resolve the exterior condition through diaphoresis.

Herba seu Flos Schizonepetae Tenuifoliae *(jing jie)* 30g
Radix Bupleuri *(chai hu)* 15g
Radix Ledebouriellae Divaricatae *(fang feng)* 10g
Herba Menthae Haplocalycis *(bo he)* 10g
Radix Codonopsitis Pilosulae *(dang shen)* 12g
Radix Astragali Membranacei *(huang qi)* 15g
Radix Angelicae Sinensis *(dang gui)* 10g
Radix Paeoniae Lactiflorae *(bai shao)* 10g
Pericarpium Citri Reticulatae *(chen pi)* 10g

MODIFICATIONS:

1. With heat associated with blood stasis due to retention, add:
   Herba Leonuri Heterophylli *(yi mu cao)* 15g
   Semen Persicae *(tao ren)* 10g
   Flos Carthami Tinctorii *(hong hua)* 10g
   Radix Salviae Miltiorrhizae *(dan shen)* 10g

2. With heat and dampness, add:
   Gypsum*(shi gao)* 6g
   Rhizoma Anemarrhenae Asphodeloidis *(zhi mu)* 12g
   Cortex Magnoliae Officinalis *(hou po)* 10g
   Rhizoma Pinelliae Ternatae *(ban xia)* 10g

ANALYSIS OF FORMULA: Radix Codonopsitis Pilosulae *(dang shen)*, Radix Astragali Membranacei *(huang qi)*, Radix Angelicae Sinensis *(dang gui),* and Radix Paeoniae Lactiflorae *(bai shao)* strengthen the qi and blood.

Herba seu Flos Schizonepetae Tenuifoliae *(jing jie)*, Radix Ledebouriellae Divaricatae *(fang feng)*, Radix Bupleuri *(chai hu)*, and Herba Menthae Haplocalycis *(bo he)* mildly release the exterior by opening the pores of the skin and promoting perspiration. Herba Leonuri Heterophylli *(yi mu cao)*, Semen Persicae *(tao ren)*, Flos Carthami Tinctorii *(hong hua)*, and Radix Salviae Miltiorrhizae *(dan shen)* remove blood stasis, especially in the genitals, as is evidenced by signs of lower abdominal pain and tenderness with a purple tongue. Some patients may also present with malodorous, purulent, and bloody lochia and a coated tongue, which are signs of heat and dampness accumulated in the lower and mid-abdomen. Rhizoma Anemarrhenae Asphodeloidis *(zhi mu)* helps Gypsum *(shi gao)* clear heat from the qi level irrespective of where it is located, in the mouth, Lungs, digestive tract, or even lower abdomen, as is the case here. Cortex Magnoliae Officinalis *(hou po)* and Rhizoma Pinelliae Ternatae *(ban xia)* resolve systemic dampness.

MECHANISM OF ACTION: A postpartum woman has a weak exterior (surface) defensive system and is therefore more vulnerable to attack by external pathogens such as wind, cold, and dampness. After such an attack the skin and muscles are said to contract, which accounts for the absence of sweating and intolerance of cold, although fever also manifests. Treatment is mainly to strengthen the exterior defensive system with qi and blood, release the muscles, and promote sweating. Since the patient can be exhausted after delivery, strong diaphoretics such as Herba Ephedrae *(ma huang)* should not be used. The mild sweat produced by the formula above dispels the pathogens without injuring the qi and blood.

Puerperal Morbidity Formula 2

STRATEGY: Nourish the vital essence, and resolve the exterior disorder.

Radix Pseudostellariae Heterophyllae *(tai zi shen)* 12g
Radix Angelicae Sinensis *(dang gui)* 9g
Tuber Ophiopogonis Japonici *(mai men dong)* 9g

Cortex Lycii Radicis *(di gu pi)* 12g

Radix Cynanchi Baiwei *(bai wei)*.. 9g

Fresh Radix Astragali Membranacei *(sheng huang qi)* 12g

Radix Rehmanniae Glutinosae *(sheng di huang)*.......................... 9g

Herba Artemisiae Annuae *(qing hao)*...................................... 9g

Carapax Amydae Sinensis *(bie jia)* 15g

Plastrum Testudinis *(gui ban)*... 15g

ANALYSIS OF FORMULA: Radix Angelicae Sinensis *(dang gui)*, Tuber Ophiopogonis Japonici *(mai men dong)*, Radix Rehmanniae Glutinosae *(sheng di huang)*, Carapax Amydae Sinensis *(bie jia)*, and Plastrum Testudinis *(gui ban)* nourish the yin. Radix Pseudostellariae Heterophyllae *(tai zi shen)* and fresh Radix Astragali Membranacei *(huang qi)* tonify the qi. Cortex Lycii Radicis *(di gu pi)*, Radix Cynanchi Baiwei *(bai wei)*, and Herba Artemisiae Annuae *(qing hao)* clear the heat which might result from yin deficiency.

MECHANISM OF ACTION: Yin deficiency can be diagnosed when patients with puerperal fever show signs of thirst, irritability, a red uncoated tongue, and a sensation of internal heat. In such cases, dispelling heat by diaphoresis may further injure the yin (vital essence). Instead, the strategy should be to nourish the yin and clear the heat with herbs that support the yin, such as Cortex Lycii Radicis *(di gu pi)*, Radix Cynanchi Baiwei *(bai wei)*, and Herba Artemisiae Annuae *(qing hao)*. Radix Astragali Membranacei *(huang qi)* and Radix Angelicae Sinensis *(dang gui)* are used together to treat or prevent anemia.

Puerperal Morbidity Formula 3

STRATEGY: Expel pathogenic heat and promote lactation.

Radix Angelicae Sinensis *(dang gui)* 9g

Radix Astragali Membranacei *(huang qi)* 12g

Herba Leonuri Heterophylli *(yi mu cao)* 12g
Cornu Cervi Degelatinatium *(lu jiao shuang)* 9g
Herba Taraxaci Mongolici cum Radice *(pu gong ying)* 12g
Fructus Arctii Lappae *(niu bang zi)* 9g
Fructus Trichosanthis *(gua lou)* 9g
Flos Lonicerae Japonicae *(jin yin hua)* 12g
Spina Gleditsiae Sinensis *(zao jiao ci)* 9g
Semen Vaccariae Segetalis *(wang bu liu xing)* 12g
Fructus Liquidambaris Taiwanianae *(lu lu tong)* 12g

ANALYSIS OF FORMULA: Cornu Cervi Degelatinatium *(lu jiao shuang)*, Fructus Trichosanthis *(gua lou)*, Fructus Arctii Lappae *(niu bang zi)*, and Spina Gleditsiae Sinensis *(zao jiao ci)* soften nodules in the breasts and assist Semen Vaccariae Segetalis *(wang bu liu xing)* and Fructus Liquid-ambaris Taiwanianae *(lu lu tong)* in promoting lactation. Herba Taraxaci Mongolici cum Radice *(pu gong ying)* and Flos Lonicerae Japonicae *(jin yin hua)* clear heat. Radix Angelicae Sinensis *(dang gui)* and Radix Astragali Membranacei *(huang qi)* tonify the qi and blood. Radix Astragali Membranacei *(huang qi)* also has the effect of increasing the flow of qi in the breast, thereby facilitating lactation.

MECHANISM OF ACTION: The painful, erythematous breast nodules are viewed as phlegm, which may produce heat if not treated in time. This is a condition of excess. After delivery the qi and blood are usually weakened, which facilitates the appearance of externally-contracted, excessive disorders. Thus Radix Astragali Membranacei *(huang qi)* and Radix Angelicae Sinensis *(dang gui)*, which are warm but not hot, and which strengthen the qi and blood, are appropriate in this case of deficiency with heat excess.

EFFICACY: In one study, 103 patients with puerperal fever were given one of the above formulas based on their respective traditional pattern diagnosis. Fever, white blood cell counts, and other signs returned to normal within eight days in all cases, and 87 patients recovered within three days.

Puerperal Thrombophlebitis

Puerperal thrombophlebitis develops mainly because of circulatory stasis, infection, or increased blood viscosity after delivery. Pelvic inflammation damages pelvic veins and initiates pelvic clotting. The incidence of pelvic thrombophlebitis is doubled in cesarean delivery as compared with vaginal delivery. Symptoms include pain, high-peaking fever, chills, and tachycardia. A tender mass may often be palpated. The lochia may be abnormal. Onset may be one week to one month after delivery or surgery. Fragmentation of the clots causes emboli to be released into the venous circulation. Large doses of antibiotics for aerobic and anaerobic organisms are needed. The patient must also remain in bed. When bacteria-infected emboli are released or when pulmonary emboli occur, heparin is indicated. Signs of pulmonary emboli include cough, blood-streaked sputum, shortness of breath, fever, and chest pain. Emboli can be seen on X-rays.

This condition is similar to the traditional disease sloughing ulcer *(tuo ju)*. The disease is caused by the attack of exogenous factors such as wind, cold, heat, and dampness into the channels while the qi and blood are weakened during the postpartum period. Obstruction in the flow of qi and blood in the channels leads to the signs and symptoms described above. Traditional Chinese medicine differentiates this disorder into two pattern-complexes: obstruction caused by damp-heat, and obstruction caused by damp-cold. Treatment is based on increasing and invigorating the flow of qi and blood, warming and clearing the channels, and removing dampness from the channels.

Herbal treatment

Thrombophlebitis Formula 1

STRATEGY: Clear the heat, invigorate the blood, remove the swelling.

Flos Lonicerae Japonicae *(jin yin hua)* 12g
Ramus Lonicerae Japonicae *(ren dong teng)* 30g
Fructus Forsythiae Suspensae *(lian qiao)* 9g

Radix Angelicae Sinensis *(dang gui)*..9g
Ramulus Sangjisheng *(sang ji sheng)*......................................15g
Radix Trichosanthis Kirilowii *(tian hua fen)*............................9g
Bulbus Fritillariae Cirrhosae *(chuan bei mu)*............................9g
Semen Benincasae Hispidae *(dong gua ren)*.............................15g

METHOD: Take daily as a decoction.

ANALYSIS OF FORMULA: Flos Lonicerae Japonicae *(jin yin hua)* and Fructus Forsythiae Suspensae *(lian qiao)* clear heat from the blood; both herbs have antibiotic properties, and are neither bitter nor so cold that they injure the Stomach. Ramus Lonicerae Japonicae *(ren dong teng)* clears heat and removes blood stasis from the channels, especially when used with Radix Angelicae Sinensis *(dang gui)*. Ramulus Sangjisheng *(sang ji sheng)* nourishes and invigorates the blood and clears the channels. Radix Trichosanthis Kirilowii *(tian hua fen)* clears heat and has the added benefit of relieving constipation. Bulbus Fritillariae Cirrhosae *(chuan bei mu)* clears heat and removes swellings due to phlegm; it also relieves pain. Semen Benincasae Hispidae *(dong gua ren)* clears heat and dampness and breaks up accumulations of phlegm.

Thrombophlebitis Formula 2

STRATEGY: Invigorate the blood, dispel blood stasis, and clear the damp-heat which is blocking the channels. (Indicated in cases where the heat is less pronounced than that for which Fomula 1 is indicated.)

Hirudo seu Whitmaniae *(shui zhi)*..6g
Tabanus *(meng chong)*...6g
Semen Persicae *(tao ren)*...6g
Radix et Rhizoma Rhei *(da huang)*..3g
Flos Lonicerae Japonicae *(jin yin hua)*...................................30g
Radix Angelicae Sinensis *(dang gui)*..9g
Radix Paeoniae Rubrae *(chi shao)*...9g
Semen Benincasae Hispidae *(dong gua ren)*.............................30g

Caulis Mutong *(mu tong)* 3g
Rhizoma Alismatis Orientalis *(ze xie)* 9g

MODIFICATION: When the symptom of reddened legs disappears, add:

Radix Astragali Membranacei *(huang qi)* 15g
Radix Codonopsitis Pilosulae *(dang shen)* 12g

ANALYSIS OF FORMULA: Hirudo seu Whitmaniae *(shui zhi)*, Tabanus *(meng chong)*, Semen Persicae *(tao ren)*, and Radix et Rhizoma Rhei *(da huang)* dissolve masses caused by blood stasis and break up swellings caused by severe blood stasis. Radix et Rhizoma Rhei *(da huang)* clears internal heat and invigorates the blood. Semen Persicae *(tao ren)*, Radix Angelicae Sinensis *(dang gui)*, and Radix Paeoniae Rubrae *(chi shao)* are used here to invigorate the blood and to cool the blood, as heat in the blood is often present in severe infections. Flos Lonicerae Japonicae *(jin yin hua)* clears internal heat. Semen Benincasae Hispidae *(dong gua ren)* clears heat and dampness, breaks up phlegm accumulations, and drains pus. Caulis Mutong *(mu tong)* and Rhizoma Alismatis Orientalis *(ze xie)* clear heat through diuresis.

DISCUSSION: In acute or subacute cases it is important to first clear the heat, dispel the blood stasis, and resolve the edema. Formula 1 addresses this phase of the disorder. When the acute symptoms abate and the fever decreases to between 37.5°C and 38°C, treatment may focus on the under-lying deficiency, which is the object of Formula 2. The second formula can also be used as an adjunct to antibiotic treatment. Treatment usually requires two to three months, with the patient remaining in bed as much as possible.

Lochiorrhea

Lochial secretions, a blood-tinged uterine discharge which includes shreds of uterine tissue and decidua, usually cease as healing completes within the fourth week postpartum. Puerperal endometritis, pelvic inflammation, retention of residual placenta, endometrial polyps, or uterine myomas can cause the subinvolution (incomplete return to its nonpregnant size) of the uterus with resulting lochiorrhea. The presentation includes fever, lower abdominal pain and tenderness, and bad-smelling lochia. Occasionally, uterine chorioepithelioma can cause postpartum uterine bleeding. If the lochial secretions do not cease within six weeks postpartum, placental retention, uterine polyps, and chorioepitheliomas should be ruled out. Antibiotics are generally used.

In traditional Chinese medicine, lochiorrhea is generally attributed to deficiency of qi and blood and uterine blood stasis. After delivery, especially during the "small full moon" (see Chapter 2), the mother needs plenty of rest and nutrition, otherwise she will not have enough qi to move and control the blood. Blood stasis of the Womb may result. Therefore, tonifying the qi and removing blood stasis is always indicated when lochiorrhea is present.

Herbal treatment

STRATEGY: Replenish the qi and blood and eliminate the blood stasis in the Womb.

Radix Codonopsitis Pilosulae *(dang shen)* 10g
Radix Astragali Membranacei *(huang qi)* 15g
Radix Angelicae Sinensis *(dang gui)* 15g
Radix Ligustici Chuanxiong *(chuan xiong)* 10g
Semen Persicae *(tao ren)* 10g
Quick-fried Rhizoma Zingiberis Officinalis *(pao jiang)* 5g
Radix Glycyrrhizae Uralensis *(gan cao)* 3g
Pollen Typhae *(pu huang)* 15g
Excrementum Trogopterori seu Pteromi *(wu ling zhi)* 10g
Folium Artemisiae Argyi *(ai ye)* 10g

METHOD: Take daily as a decoction.

MODIFICATIONS:

1. When blood stasis is apparent, add:
   Herba Leonuri Heterophylli *(yi mu cao)* 12g

2. When qi and blood deficiency is apparent, add:

Rhizoma Atractylodis Macrocephalae *(bai zhu)* 9g

Radix Rehmanniae Glutinosae Conquitae *(shu di huang)* 12g

Gelatinum Corii Asini *(e jiao)* 9g

3. With heat and blood stasis, add:

Cortex Moutan Radicis *(mu dan pi)* 9g

Herba cum Radice Patriniae *(bai jiang cao)* 30g

Herba Taraxaci Mongolici cum Radice *(pu gong ying)* 30g

Herba cum Radice Violae Yedoensitis *(zi hua di ding)* 15g

Herba Hedyotidis Diffusae *(bai hua she she cao)* 30g

4. With yin deficiency and internal heat, omit the quick-fried Rhizoma Zingiberis Officinalis *(pao jiang),* and add:

Cortex Moutan Radicis *(mu dan pi)* 9g

Radix Scrophulariae Ningpoensis *(xuan shen)* 9g

ANALYSIS OF FORMULA: Radix Codonopsitis Pilosulae *(dang shen),* Radix Astragali Membranacei *(huang qi),* and Rhizoma Atractylodis Macro-cephalae *(bai zhu)* are used to tonify the qi, while Radix Angelicae Sinensis *(dang gui)* and Radix Rehmanniae Glutinosae Conquitae *(shu di huang)* tonify the blood. Radix Astragali Membranacei *(huang qi)* and Radix Angelicae Sinensis *(dang gui)* are always used together when tonifying the blood. Semen Persicae *(tao ren),* Radix Ligustici Chuanxiong *(chuan xiong),* Pollen Typhae *(pu huang),* Excrementum Trogopterori seu Pteromi *(wu ling zhi),* and Herba Leonuri Heterophylli *(yi mu cao)* invigorate the blood and remove stasis. Ginger, in its quick-fried form, loses its pungent properties, but remains effective in expelling local cold that causes qi and blood stagnation. Quick-fried Rhizoma Zingiberis Officinalis *(pao jiang)* is black in color. According to the five-phase theory, it will stop bleeding, since water checks fire, and black checks red. If heat results from yin defi-ciency, baked ginger is often omitted from the formula because it is so warm. Folium Artemisiae Argyi *(ai ye)* is less warm and gently expels the cold—which causes stagnation of qi and blood—from the Womb and channels. Cortex Moutan Radicis *(mu dan pi)* and Radix Scrophulariae

Ningpoensis *(xuan shen)* cool the internal heat associated with yin deficiency. Herba cum Radice Patriniae *(bai jiang cao)*, Herba Taraxaci Mongolici cum Radice *(pu gong ying)*, Herba Hedyotidis Diffusae *(bai hua she she cao)*, and Herba cum Radice Violae Yedoensitis *(zi hua di ding)* clear the internal heat associated with excess.

EFFICACY: In one study of 23 patients with puerperal lochiorrhea, 21 patients (91%) were cured using this formula. The remaining two cases required antibiotics to be cured. Sixteen patients (70%) were cured within three days, four were cured within six days, and the remaining three patients were cured in an average of ten days.

Acute Mastitis

Mastitis occurs most frequently in primiparous nursing mothers, and is usually caused by the coagulase-positive *Staphylococcus aureus* entering through a fissure or a duct. Inflammation of the breast seldom occurs before the fifth day after delivery. The infection may be limited to the subareolar region, but more frequently involves an obstructed lactiferous duct and the surrounding parenchyma. Many infants harbor infections and infect the mother's breast during nursing. Signs and symptoms are malaise, unilateral breast tenderness, and temperature peaks of 39-40°C (102-104°F). The breast is reddened over the infected area, exquisitely tender, and indurated. Most commonly a painful erythematous lobule in the outer quadrant is noted during the second or third week postpartum. In the presence of acute mastitis, it is best to discontinue nursing and to apply local heat (or cold), use a well-fitted brassiere, and institute appropriate antibiotic treatment. If the infection is not treated properly, a breast abcess may develop. Pitting edema over the site of inflammation and some degree of fluctuation are signs of abcess formation. In these cases, incision or opening of the loculated areas with wide drainage is necessary.

In traditional Chinese medicine, the Stomach channel traverses the breasts and the nipple connects to the Liver channel. Stagnancy of the Liver and intense heat in the Stomach as are found in postpartum women interfere with nursing. Mastitis occurs when an external pathogen invades the breast. The traditional diagnosis is therefore one of pathogenic fire invasion due to stagnancy in the breast and its related channels, leading to heat from constraint and nodules in the breast.

Herbal treatment

Mastitis Formula 1

STRATEGY: Eliminate the toxic heat, soften the nodules, and promote lactation.

Herba Taraxaci Mongolici cum Radice *(pu gong ying)*..................60g

Flos Lonicerae Japonicae *(jin yin hua)*....................................30g

Fructus Forsythiae Suspensae *(lian qiao)*..................................15g

Fructus Trichosanthis *(gua lou)*...20g

Bulbus Fritillariae Thunbergii *(zhe bei mu)*..............................12g

Gummi Olibanum *(ru xiang)*..10g

Myrrha *(mo yao)*..10g

Spina Gleditsiae Sinensis *(zao jiao ci)*...................................15g

Squama Manitis Pentadactylae *(chuan shan jia)*.........................10g

Radix Paeoniae Rubrae *(chi shao)*..15g

METHOD: Take daily as a decoction.

MODIFICATIONS:

1. With high fever, add:
   Herba cum Radice Houttuyniae Cordatae *(yu xing cao)*..............30g
   Herba cum Radice Violae Yedoensitis *(zi hua di ding)*...............15g
   Fructus Gardeniae Jasminoidis *(zhi zi)*................................12g

2. With insufficient lactation, add:
   Nidus Vespae *(lu feng fang)*...12g
   Fructus Liquidambaris Taiwanianae *(lu lu tong)*......................15g

3. Blood stasis is present when breast nodules can be palpated and there
is low fever. In such cases, add:

Rhizoma Sparganii Stoloniferi *(san leng)*..................................9g

Rhizoma Curcumae Ezhu *(e zhu)*..9g

ANALYSIS OF FORMULA: Herba Taraxaci Mongolici cum Radice *(pu gong ying)*, Herba cum Radice Houttuyniae Cordatae *(yu xing cao)*, and Herba cum Radice Violae Yedoensitis *(zi hua di ding)* reduce heat and local swelling. Fructus Forsythiae Suspensae *(lian qiao)* and Flos Lonicerae Japonicae *(jin yin hua)* eliminate toxic heat. Fructus Gardeniae Jasminoidis *(zhi zi)* expels heat from the Liver channel. Radix Paeoniae Rubrae *(chi shao)*, Fructus Trichosanthis *(gua lou)*, Gummi Olibanum *(ru xiang)*, and Myrrha*(mo yao)* break up nodules and remove blood stasis in order to relieve the pain. Squama Manitis Pentadactylae *(chuan shan jia)*, Spina Gleditsiae Sinensis *(zao jiao ci)*, and Bulbus Fritillariae Thunbergii *(zhe bei mu)* dissolve nodules and clear the heat. Nidus Vespae *(lu feng fang)* and Fructus Liquidambaris Taiwanianae *(lu lu tong)* are used to guide the actions of the formula to the breast and through the Liver channel. Rhizoma Sparganii Stoloniferi *(san leng)* and Rhizoma Curcumae Ezhu *(e zhu)* break up the nodules. In addition, Rhizoma Sparganii Stoloniferi *(san leng)* breaks up "stagnant qi within the blood," while Rhizoma Curcumae Ezhu *(e zhu)* breaks up "congealed blood within the qi."

MECHANISM OF ACTION: No mechanism of action has been proposed for this formula.

EFFICACY: In a study of 40 patients treated for mastitis with this formula in combination with antibiotics, 26 were cured within three days, and the remaining 14 were cured within six days.

Mastitis Formula 2

STRATEGY: Soothe the Liver, resolve the phlegm, and promote lactation. This formula is used mainly for subacute cases.

Spina Gleditsiae Sinensis *(zao jiao ci)* 90g

Radix Bupleuri *(chai hu)* 10g

Radix Paeoniae Lactiflorae *(bai shao)* 10g

Radix Glycyrrhizae Uralensis *(gan cao)* 6g

METHOD: Take daily as a decoction.

ANALYSIS OF FORMULA: Spina Gleditsiae Sinensis *(zao jiao ci)*, the for-mula's principal herb, invigorates the blood, reduces swelling, dissolves nodes, and promotes lactation when used in large doses. Radix Bupleuri *(chai hu)* soothes the Liver and helps the flow of qi. Radix Paeoniae Lactiflorae *(bai shao)* nourishes the yin of the Liver, soothes the Liver, har-monizes the blood, and relieves pain. Radix Glycyrrhizae Uralensis *(gan cao)* is used in general for its ability to relieve toxicity, and here specifically to relieve the toxic fever.

MECHANISM OF ACTION: This formula increases the level of an immune substance, complement 3 (C3), which helps combat the infection. Other mechanisms are probable but have yet to be identified.

EFFICACY: In a study of 36 mastitis patients treated with the above for-mula and without antibiotics, 17 were cured within seven days, while 19 were cured after local drainage in addition to the herbal treatment.

Mastitis Formula 3

STRATEGY: Clear the heat, invigorate the blood, and reduce the swelling.

Mirabilitum *(mang xiao)* 250g

Radix et Rhizoma Rhei *(da huang)* 25g

METHOD: Break up the Mirabilitum *(mang xiao)* and grind the Radix et Rhizoma Rhei *(da huang)* into a powder. Mix the two ingredients and put them into a cloth bag. Bind the bag tightly to the affected breast and keep it there for 12 hours. This method is contraindicated if there is a ruptured abcess or an ulcer.

ANALYSIS OF FORMULA: Mirabilitum *(mang xiao)* is said to draw out the fluids in order to drain the swelling. Powdered Radix et Rhizoma Rhei *(da huang)* penetrates the skin, invigorates the blood, and clears the heat. This formula is often used in conjunction with an oral decoction.

9

Miscellaneous Conditions

Postmenopausal Syndrome and Osteoporosis

POSTMENOPAUSAL SYNDROME CONSISTS of a broad range of symptoms associated with the regression of ovarian function around the time of menopause. These symptoms are mainly related to instability of the autonomic nervous system: hot flashes, perspiration, irritability, dizziness, itching, depression, anxiety, memory loss, decrease in breast size, palpitations, and frequent or urgent urination. During the three years that follow, bone loss is quite pronounced, thus osteoporosis is the most important health hazard associated with menopause. Vertebral bodies are the most common sites of fracture, and Colles', hip, and other fractures have a very high incidence as well.

The basic cause of postmenopausal syndrome is a considerable drop in estrogen level, which affects the neuroendocrine and immune systems and is responsible for bone loss. Estrogen alone or in combination with progesterone or testosterone is the treatment of choice in spite of the continuing controversy regarding the increased risk of endometrial or breast cancer. Adding progesterone or testosterone reduces the risk of malignancy. Prevention of osteoporosis is the major reason to be weighed against those risks.

The traditional literature relates that women's Kidneys begin to fade from the age of thirty-five. Heavenly dew *(tian gui)*, the ovaries and their function, are exhausted by age forty-nine. All the symptoms associated with post-menopausal syndrome can be explained in terms of the loss of Kidney yin, leading to a deficiency of Liver or Heart yin, which then transforms into Liver or Heart fire and internal heat. Sometimes the Kidney yang becomes deficient also, and qi deficiency results, which can lead to blood stasis. The Kidneys nourish the brain, bones, and bone marrow. This further explains the derivation of the symptoms, particularly the loss of bone.

Herbal treatment

STRATEGY: Strengthen the Kidneys and Liver, extinguish Liver fire, and clear the heat. The object of this treatment is not only to relieve the symptoms, but also to delay the onset of senility and to increase the lifespan.

Menopause Formula 1

Herba Epimedii *(yin yang huo)* 15g
Honey-toasted Radix Glycyrrhizae Uralensis *(zhi gan cao)*...............6g
Semen Tritici Aestivi Levis *(fu xiao mai)* 30g
Fructus Zizyphi Jujubae *(da zao)* 6g
Radix Bupleuri *(chai hu)*...9g
Fructus Gardeniae Jasminoidis *(zhi zi)*....................................9g
Ginger-prepared Rhizoma Pinelliae Ternatae *(jiang ban xia)* 9g
Radix Scutellariae Baicalensis *(huang qin)* 9g
Radix Codonopsitis Pilosulae *(dang shen)*................................12g
Concha Margaritaferae *(zhen zhu mu)* 30g

METHOD: Take daily as a decoction for three months.

MODIFICATIONS:

1. With hypertension, add:
   Ramulus cum Uncis Uncariae *(gou teng)* 15g
   Lumbricus *(di long)* 9g
   Radix Achyranthis Bidentatae *(niu xi)* 9g

2. With insomnia, add:
   Fructus Schisandrae Chinensis *(wu wei zi)* 3g
   Caulis Polygoni Multiflori *(ye jiao teng)* 15g

3. With thirst, add:
   Herba Dendrobii *(shi hu)* 12g
   Rhizoma Polygonati Odorati *(yu zhu)* 9g

ANALYSIS OF FORMULA: This combination is effective in controlling hot flashes, perspiration, and depression. Herba Epimedii *(yin yang huo)* is the chief herb for tonifying both the Kidney yin and yang. Radix Bupleuri *(chai hu)*, Radix Codonopsitis Pilosulae *(dang shen)*, ginger-prepared Rhizoma Pinelliae Ternatae *(jiang ban xia)*, honey-toasted Radix Glycyrrhizae Uralensis *(zhi gan cao),* and Radix Scutellariae Baicalensis *(huang qin)* are an integral part of the classical formula Minor Bupleurum Decoction *(xiao chai hu tang)*. Here they are used to relieve symptoms associated with Liver obstruction, such as depression and anxiety. Semen Tritici Aestivi Levis *(fu xiao mai)* and Fructus Zizyphi Jujubae *(da zao)* benefit the Heart and reduce anxiety. Fructus Gardeniae Jasminoidis *(zhi zi)* clears Liver fire and is used to calm irritability. Concha Margaritaferae *(zhen zhu mu)* is used as a sedative.

MECHANISM OF ACTION: This treatment is empirical and seems to provide good symptomatic relief. No experimental data is available to explain the mechanism.

EFFICACY: In a study of 43 women treated for postmenopausal syndrome, 19 obtained complete relief of their symptoms, and another 19 obtained marked improvement, for a total rate of effectiveness of about 86%.

Menopause Formula 2

Radix Rehmanniae Glutinosae *(sheng di huang)* 15g
Radix Paeoniae Lactiflorae *(bai shao)* 12g
Fructus Lycii *(gou qi zi)* 12g
Plastrum Testudinis *(gui ban)* 18g
Herba Epimedii *(yin yang huo)* 12g
Radix Morindae Officinalis *(ba ji tian)* 12g
Herba Cistanches *(rou cong rong)* 12g
Rhizoma Anemarrhenae Asphodeloidis *(zhi mu)* 15g
Radix Scutellariae Baicalensis *(huang qin)* 9g
Rhizoma Coptidis *(huang lian)* 3g
Sclerotium Poriae Cocos *(fu ling)* 9g

METHOD: Take daily as a decoction for three months.

ANALYSIS OF FORMULA: Radix Rehmanniae Glutinosae *(sheng di huang),* Radix Paeoniae Lactiflorae *(bai shao),* Fructus Lycii *(gou qi zi),* and Plastrum Testudinis *(gui ban)* are used to replenish the yin of the Kidneys and Liver. Herba Epimedii *(yin yang huo),* Radix Morindae Officinalis *(ba ji tian),* and Herba Cistanches *(rou cong rong)* support the Kidney yang in accordance with the principle, "When tonifying the yin, tonify the yang as well." The Kidneys are responsible for the essence and are closely related to the bones, hair, brain, and reproductive system, thus the emphasis on the Kidneys. Rhizoma Anemarrhenae Asphodeloidis *(zhi mu)* clears internal heat caused by Kidney yin deficiency, while Radix Scutellariae Baicalensis *(huang qin)* clears Liver fire, Rhizoma Coptidis *(huang lian)* clears Heart fire, and Sclerotium Poriae Cocos *(fu ling)* removes Heart fire through the urine.

EFFICACY: In a study of 22 women treated with the above formula, six experienced relief from all symptoms and 12 showed marked improvement, for a total rate of effectiveness of 82%. Two other women showed slight improvement.

MECHANISM OF ACTION: Data show that endogenous estrogen levels are lower in postmenopausal women with postmenopausal syndrome than in postmenopausal women without the syndrome. After treatment, their estrogen levels rose to levels comparable to symptom-free postmenopausal women. Herbs in the formula also help regulate the immune system and central transmitters such as endorphins, 5-HT, and norepinephrine. Peripheral T-helper cell counts and interleukin-2 levels are significantly increased as well. These results may explain how the Kidneys are involved in neuroendocrine and immune regulation, and perhaps in calcium regulation and bone loss, in postmenopausal women.

Urinary Incontinence

Incontinence may be associated with stress, may occur without stress (true incontinence), or it may be due to infection, neuro-vesical disease (urgency), or overflow of urine. Stress incontinence occurs when the patient is standing, usually postpartum or as a result of relaxation of the pelvic floor (connective tissues, fascia, and muscles). Most senile incontinence is due to disorders of the neuro-vesical center. Treatment may be difficult and often requires urologic consultation.

In traditional Chinese medicine, most urinary incontinence is attributed to cold in the Lower Burner. Herbs or acupuncture can be used to warm the Lower Burner. Exercises that strengthen the anal levator muscle can also be helpful.

Herbal treatment

STRATEGY: Tonify the Lower Burner in order to control the urine.

Fructus Alpiniae Oxyphyllae *(yi zhi ren)* 12g
Radix Linderae Strychnifoliae *(wu yao)* 9g
Radix Dioscoreae Oppositae *(shan yao)* 12g

MODIFICATIONS:

1. With a sensation of pulling down, add:
   Radix Codonopsitis Pilosulae *(dang shen)* 12g

Rhizoma Atractylodis Macrocephalae *(bai zhu)* 9g
Rhizoma Cimicifugae *(sheng ma)* 9g

2. With dark urine and dysuria, add:
Rhizoma Coptidis *(huang lian)* 3g
Herba Lophatheri Gracilis *(dan zhu ye)* 9g
Tips of Radix Glycyrrhizae Uralensis *(gan cao shao)* 6g

ANALYSIS OF FORMULA: Fructus Alpiniae Oxyphyllae *(yi zhi ren)* and
Radix Dioscoreae Oppositae *(shan yao)* tonify the Spleen and Kidneys and
strengthen the Bladder. Radix Linderae Strychnifoliae *(wu yao)* warms the
Kidneys and promotes the flow of qi in the Lower Burner (it is often used
to relieve pain). Radix Codonopsitis Pilosulae *(dang shen)*, Rhizoma
Atractylodis Macrocephalae *(bai zhu)*, and Rhizoma Cimicifugae *(sheng
ma)* augment and raise the qi in order to retain the urine. Rhizoma
Coptidis *(huang lian)* expels heat from the Heart. Herba Lophatheri
Gracilis *(dan zhu ye)* clears heat from the Heart by way of diuresis through
the Small Intestine, which is the paired Organ of the Heart. The Small
Intestine's function is to separate the waste from what is useful; it rids the
waste through the Bladder and Large Intestine. This association is therefore quite useful in draining heat from the Bladder. The tips of Radix
Glycyrrhizae Uralensis *(gan cao shao)* clear fire from the urethra. This formula is a popular remedy drawn from the traditional literature, and is
known as Guide Out the Red Powder *(dao chi san)*. It has a long history,
and its efficacy in treating incontinence is time-tested.

MECHANISM OF ACTION: The mechanism of action of this formula has yet
to be explained.

Acupuncture treatment

STRATEGY: Warm the Lower Burner and regulate urination.

CV-4 *(guan yuan)*
CV-3 *(zhong ji)*
GV-4 *(ming men)*
BL-23 *(shen shu)*

METHOD: Treat daily, retaining the needles for 30 minutes while warming them with moxa. Ten days constitute a course of treatment.

ANALYSIS OF FORMULA: The Conception and Governing vessels, together with the lower trunk part of the Bladder channel, are closely associated with urogenital function. A detailed mechanism of action has yet to be identified.

Uterine Myoma

About 35% of all women over age 35 have myomas. The majority of myomas are benign and cause no symptoms. Malignancy occurs in less than 0.5% of cases. Uterine myomas may occur as an isolated growth, but are more likely to be multiple and of varied size. The patient's initial complaint may be infertility. There may also be menorrhagia or abnormal endometrial bleeding in case of interstitial or submucous myoma. Symptoms due to pressure on the neighboring organs may also be present. Uncommon symptoms such as pain may be the result of degeneration or expulsion of the myoma. In most instances, myomas do not require treatment, particularly if there are no symptoms or if the patient is postmenopausal. Surgery is indicated when the myoma gives the appearance of more than twelve weeks of pregnancy. Hormonal therapy for shrinking the mass has been reported, but hormones must be used with caution and the size of the tumor must be followed up closely. Before any treatment, an endometrial pathological study is necessary to rule out malignancy.

In traditional Chinese medicine a myoma is regarded simply as a "uterine mass" caused by stagnancy of qi and blood and by obstruction of the Womb due to phlegm and heat. The pathogenesis of menorrhagia, pain, and mass are fully accounted for by this model.

Herbal treatment

STRATEGY: Promote the flow of qi and blood, soften the mass, and break up the accumulation of phlegm.

Radix Astragali Membranacei *(huang qi)* 30g

Radix Codonopsitis Pilosulae *(dang shen)* 10g

Rhizoma Sparganii Stoloniferi *(san leng)* 10g

Rhizoma Curcumae Ezhu *(e zhu)*. 10g

Rhizoma Cyperi Rotundi *(xiang fu)*. 10g

Semen Persicae *(tao ren)* 10g

Flos Carthami Tinctorii *(hong hua)* 10g

Radix Angelicae Sinensis *(dang gui)*. 10g

Thallus Algae *(kun bu)* 10g

Squama Manitis Pentadactylae *(chuan shan jia)* 10g

Spica Prunellae Vulgaris *(xia ku cao)*. 10g

Semen Vaccariae Segetalis *(wang bu liu xing)* 10g

METHOD: Take daily as a decoction.

MODIFICATIONS:

1. With heavy bleeding, omit Flos Carthami Tinctorii *(hong hua)* and
   Radix Angelicae Sinensis *(dang gui)*, and add:
   Radix Notoginseng *(san qi)*. 5g
   Os Draconis *(long gu)*. 18g
   Concha Ostreae *(mu li)* 18g
   Os Sepiae seu Sepiellae *(hai piao xiao)*. 12g
   Radix Rubiae Cordifoliae *(qian cao gen)* 12g
   Gelatinum Corii Asini *(e jiao)*. 9g

2. With cold in the lower abdomen, add:
   Fructus Evodiae Rutaecarpae *(wu zhu yu)*. 10g
   Fructus Foeniculi Vulgaris *(xiao hui xiang)* 5g
   Cortex Cinnamomi Cassiae *(rou gui)*. 3g

3. With insomnia, add:
   Caulis Polygoni Multiflori *(ye jiao teng)*. 12g
   Radix Polygalae Tenuifoliae *(yuan zhi)*. 10g
   Semen Zizyphi Spinosae *(suan zao ren)*. 20g

ANALYSIS OF FORMULA: Radix Astragali Membranacei *(huang qi)* and Radix Codonopsitis Pilosulae *(dang shen)* tonify the qi and promote its flow. In case of myoma with heavy bleeding, it is also necessary to tonify the blood. Radix Angelicae Sinensis *(dang gui)* and Gelatinum Corii Asini *(e jiao)* are included for this purpose. Flos Carthami Tinctorii *(hong hua)*, Semen Persicae *(tao ren)*, Radix Angelicae Sinensis *(dang gui)*, Rhizoma Sparganii Stoloniferi *(san leng)*, Radix Notoginseng *(san qi)*, and Radix Rubiae Cordifoliae *(qian cao gen)* invigorate the blood. Rhizoma Curcumae Ezhu *(e zhu)* and Rhizoma Cyperi Rotundi *(xiang fu)* regulate the flow of qi and blood. Thallus Algae *(kun bu)*, Squama Manitis Pentadactylae *(chuan shan jia)*, Spica Prunellae Vulgaris *(xia ku cao)*, Os Draconis *(long gu)*, and Concha Ostreae *(mu li)* clear heat, soften masses, and dissolve phlegm. Os Sepiae seu Sepiellae *(hai piao xiao)* and Gelatinum Corii Asini *(e jiao)* stop bleeding. Fructus Evodiae Rutaecarpae *(wu zhu yu)*, Fructus Foeniculi Vulgaris *(xiao hui xiang)*, and Cortex Cinnamomi Cassiae *(rou gui)* warm the lower abdomen, promote the flow of qi and blood, and dispel cold. Caulis Polygoni Multiflori *(ye jiao teng)*, Radix Polygalae Tenuifoliae *(yuan zhi)*, and Semen Zizyphi Spinosae *(suan zao ren)* treat insomnia, and are especially useful for blood deficiency.

MECHANISM OF ACTION: None has been proposed.

EFFICACY: The efficacy of this treatment varies. In one study, the formula was given to 41 patients whose myomas gave the appearance of a uterus less than eight weeks pregnant. Nine showed a significant reduction in size of the mass, 14 showed improvement, while 18 experienced little or no effect.

Uterine Prolapse

Uterine prolapse is the abnormal protrusion of the uterus through the pelvic floor aperture or genital hiatus. It occurs most commonly multiparae as a result of progressive injury to the endopelvic muscles and fascia caused by childbirth. Uterine prolapse may also be the result of pelvic tumor, chronic bronchitis, or other mechanical cause. A vaginal pessary may be used as a palliative in mild or moderate cases. Vaginal hysterectomy with anteroposterior colpoperinerrhaphy provides excellent and permanent results, but this surgery is commonly postponed until after the childbearing age.

Traditional Chinese medicine regards uterine prolapse as an injury due to childbirth. Since the Spleen is associated with the muscles and the qi, and the Kidneys with the Womb, vulva, and urethra, uterine prolapse can be related to deficiency of the Spleen or of the Kidneys.

Herbal treatment

STRATEGY: Raise the qi in order to lift the uterus back in place.

Radix Codonopsitis Pilosulae *(dang shen)* 15g
Radix Astragali Membranacei *(huang qi)* 15g
Rhizoma Cimicifugae *(sheng ma)* 9g
Rhizoma Atractylodis Macrocephalae *(bai zhu)* 15g
Rhizoma Polygonati *(huang jing)* 15g
Plastrum Testudinis *(gui ban)* 15g
Fructus Citri Aurantii *(zhi ke)* 20g
Radix Morindae Officinalis *(ba ji tian)* 20g
Radix Angelicae Sinensis *(dang gui)* 9g
Herba Leonuri Heterophylli *(yi mu cao)* 30g

METHOD: Take daily as a decoction, in combination with the following topical formula:

Herba Leonuri Heterophylli *(yi mu cao)* 30g
Fructus Citri Aurantii *(zhi ke)* 30g

METHOD: Boil the herbs and steam the perineum, then use as a sitz bath for 15 minutes each day.

ANALYSIS OF FORMULA: Radix Codonopsitis Pilosulae *(dang shen)*, Radix Astragali Membranacei *(huang qi)*, Rhizoma Atractylodis Macrocephalae *(bai zhu)*, and Rhizoma Cimicifugae *(sheng ma)* raise the qi and lift prolapsed organs. Fructus Citri Aurantii *(zhi ke)* and Herba

Leonuri Heterophylli *(yi mu cao)*, in large doses only, make the uterine muscle contract. Rhizoma Polygonati *(huang jing)* and Radix Morindae Officinalis *(ba ji tian)* tonify the Kidneys.

EFFICACY: In a study of 20 patients with mild or moderate prolapse, 15 were relieved of symptoms, while the remaining five experienced some improvement but were not cured.

Acupuncture treatment

STRATEGY: Tonify the Kidneys and invigorate the qi to lift the prolapsed organ back in place.

CV-3 *(zhong ji)*
CV-1 *(hui yin)*
GV-20 *(bai hui)*
GB-26 *(dai mai)*
SP-6 *(san yin jiao)*

METHOD: Treat every other day, retaining the needles for 30 minutes, and warming the needle at GV-20 *(bai hui)* with moxa. Ten treatments constitute a course.

MODIFICATION: With cold, needle and use moxa at BL-21 *(wei shu)* and BL-23 *(shen shu)*.

EXPLANATION OF POINTS: Acupuncture is to be used as an adjunct treatment only. GV-20 *(bai hui)* raises the qi and lifts prolapsed organs. GB-26 *(dai mai)* connects with the Girdle vessel *(dai mai)*, which controls the channels that cross the waist, and is thus helpful when the uterus is prolapsed. CV-1 *(hui yin)* and CV-3 *(zhong ji)* strengthen the muscles of the reproductive tract. CV-3 *(zhong ji)*, SP-6 *(san yin jiao)*, BL-21 *(wei shu)*, and BL-23 *(shen shu)* tonify the Spleen and Kidneys.

EFFICACY: Temporary improvement has been reported using this method. It is usually combined with one of the herbal treatments described above.

Fibrocystic Breast Disease

Fibrocystic breast disease is also known as chronic cystic mastitis or cystic hyperplasia of the breast. It is common in women between 30 and 50 years of age, but rare in postmenopausal women. This suggests that etiology of this disorder is related to ovarian function. The disorder may manifest as asymptomatic lumps in the breast, but pain and tenderness often call attention to the mass at the premenstrual phase of the cycle, at which time the cysts tend to enlarge. Symptoms disappear when the menses start. Cyclic breast pain and size variation, and the multiplicity of lesions, are most helpful in differentiating the disease from carcinoma. Definitive diagnosis often relies on biopsy. Wearing a brassiere is recommended for protection and support and to avoid trauma. Bromocryptine may relieve the pain, but hormone therapy is not advisable because of undesirable side effects.

In traditional Chinese medicine, the breast is associated with the Liver and the Spleen. Fibrocystic breast disease is regarded as "premenstrual breast engorgement," attributable to stagnancy of the Liver due to constrained emotions. Too much stagnancy in the Liver weakens the Spleen, which is then unable to regulate the flow of water. Water accumulates in the breasts as phlegm. If there is Liver fire, patients will also complain of thirst and premenstrual irritability, and the pulse will be wiry.

Herbal treatment

Fibrocystic Formula 1

STRATEGY: Remove Liver stagnancy, break up the mass, invigorate the blood.

Fructus Hordei Vulgaris Germinantus *(mai ya)* 30-60g
Fructus Crataegi *(shan zha)* 20g
Spica Prunellae Vulgaris *(xia ku cao)* 20g
Radix et Caulis Jixueteng *(ji xue teng)* 30g
Concha Ostreae *(mu li)* 30g

Carapax Amydae Sinensis *(bie jia)* 30g
Radix Paeoniae Rubrae *(chi shao)* 15g
Radix Salviae Miltiorrhizae *(dan shen)*. 15g
Pericarpium Citri Reticulatae *(chen pi)* 10g
Medulla Tetrapanacis Papyriferi *(tong cao)* 10g
Rhizoma Sparganii Stoloniferi *(san leng)* 12g
Rhizoma Curcumae Ezhu *(e zhu)*. 12g

METHOD: Take daily as a decoction, except during menses, for three menstrual cycles.

MODIFICATIONS:

1. With qi deficiency, add:
   Radix Codonopsitis Pilosulae *(dang shen)* 12g
   Radix Astragali Membranacei *(huang qi)* 12g
   Radix Angelicae Sinensis *(dang gui)*. 12g

2. With heavy breast engorgement, add:
   Fructus Meliae Toosendan *(chuan lian zi)* 12g
   Rhizoma Corydalis Yanhusuo *(yan hu suo)*. 12g
   Cortex Moutan Radicis *(mu dan pi)* 9g
   Fructus Gardeniae Jasminoidis *(zhi zi)*. 12g

ANALYSIS OF FORMULA: Fructus Hordei Vulgaris Germinantus *(mai ya)* removes food stagnation, restrains lactation, and disperses breast masses. Concha Ostreae *(mu li)*, Carapax Amydae Sinensis *(bie jia)*, Fructus Crataegi *(shan zha)*, Rhizoma Curcumae Ezhu *(e zhu),* and Rhizoma Sparganii Stoloniferi *(san leng)* soften and disperse hard lumps. Non-calcined Concha Ostreae *(mu li)* is used to soften and disperse; it is calcined to enrich the yin and to sedate. Spica Prunellae Vulgaris *(xia ku cao)* and Pericarpium Citri Reticulatae *(chen pi)* move the Liver qi. Radix et Caulis Jixueteng *(ji xue teng)*, Radix Paeoniae Rubrae *(chi shao),* and Radix Salviae Miltiorrhizae *(dan shen)* invigorate the blood. Medulla Tetrapanacis Papyriferi *(tong cao)* is used to drain water from the breast and thus reduce the size of the nodules. It also promotes lactation and thus counteracts the prolactin-lowering action of Fructus Hordei Vulgaris Germinantus *(mai ya)*.

REMARK: Either Pericarpium Citri Reticulatae *(chen pi)* or Pericarpium Citri Reticulatae Viride *(qing pi)* may be used in this formula. Pericarpium Citri Reticulatae *(chen pi)* is mild and treats the Lungs and the Spleen; Pericarpium Citri Reticulatae Viride *(qing pi)* is dry and more potent, and helps the flow of Liver qi. Since most of the herbs in this formula are quite strong, it is sufficient to use Pericarpium Citri Reticulatae *(chen pi)* to help the flow of qi without risk that this will dry the patient's fluids. If the patient's yin is strong, Pericarpium Citri Reticulatae Viride *(qing pi)* may be substituted.

MECHANISM OF ACTION: The mechanism of action has yet to be identified.

EFFICACY: In a study of 54 women with mammary dysplasia who were treated with this formula, 36 were completely relieved of symptoms and their breast lumps disappeared. Eleven saw their symptoms and breast lumps reduced by half, five experienced relapses, and two saw no change in symptoms.

Fibrocystic Formula 2

STRATEGY: Invigorate the blood and soften the lumps.

Cornu Cervi *(lu jiao)* 15g
Squama Manitis Pentadactylae *(chuan shan jia)* 9g
Rhizoma Sparganii Stoloniferi *(san leng)* 9g
Rhizoma Curcumae Ezhu *(e zhu)* 9g
Radix Salviae Miltiorrhizae *(dan shen)* 15g
Radix Angelicae Sinensis *(dang gui)* 12g
Myrrha*(mo yao)* 10g
Rhizoma Corydalis Yanhusuo *(yan hu suo)* 10g
Herba Epimedii *(yin yang huo)* 10g

Concha Ostreae *(mu li)* 10g

Radix Astragali Membranacei *(huang qi)* 20g

METHOD: Take daily as a decoction.

ANALYSIS OF FORMULA: Rhizoma Sparganii Stoloniferi *(san leng)*, Rhizoma Curcumae Ezhu *(e zhu)*, Radix Angelicae Sinensis *(dang gui)*, Radix Salviae Miltiorrhizae *(dan shen)*, and Concha Ostreae *(mu li)* invigorate the blood and soften lumps. Squama Manitis Pentadactylae *(chuan shan jia)* breaks up hard lumps. Cornu Cervi *(lu jiao)* is also effective in reducing breast masses and treating deep-rooted carbuncles, in addition to its better-known function of tonifying the Kidney yang. Myrrha *(mo yao)* and Rhizoma Corydalis Yanhusuo *(yan hu suo)* promote the flow of qi and blood. Radix Astragali Membranacei *(huang qi)* helps the flow of qi and thereby facilitates the removal of water. Herba Epimedii *(yin yang huo)* tonifies the Kidneys in order to regulate the menstrual cycle.

MECHANISM OF ACTION: The mechanism of action has yet to be identified.

EFFICACY: In a study of 50 patients treated with this formula for 60 days, 19 were cured and mammography showed a complete resolution of their breast lumps, while the remaining 31 saw a reduction in the size of the mass.

Acupuncture treatment

STRATEGY: Promote the flow of qi in the Liver channel, and expel heat and water.

Method 1

ST-15 *(wu yi)*

CV-17 *(shan zhong)*

LI-4 *(he gu)*

Method 2

SI-11 *(tian zong)*
GB-21 *(jian jing)*
BL-18 *(gan shu)*

METHOD: Treat daily, alternating the two formulas every other day.

ANALYSIS OF FORMULA: The Stomach channel traverses the breasts, and the Liver channel connects to the the nipple and breast. ST-15 *(wu yi)* is a local point that is used to promote the local flow of qi as a means of reducing the nodules. CV-17 *(shan zhong)* is the influential point of the qi, which is commonly used to promote the flow of qi in the chest. As a major yang brightness point, LI-4 *(he gu)* is used to treat areas of both the chest and head that are traversed by yang brightness channels.

SI-11 *(tian zong)* is a point that has the special function of treating a variety of breast disorders. Because of the Gallbladder channel's inner/outer relationship with the Liver channel, points on the Gallbladder channel can also be used to clear heat from the Liver channel. This, in part, explains the function of GB-21 *(jian jing)* in clearing heat from the breast via the Liver channel's relationship to the breast. BL-18 *(gan shu)* is the associated point of the Liver channel and is needled to invigorate the flow of qi in the Liver channel.

MECHANISM OF ACTION: Following acupuncture treatment, the serum E_2 level decreases while the progesterone level increases. This suggests regulation of the hormone ratio. The mechanism is not fully explained.

EFFICACY: In a study of 500 patients treated at irregular intervals (not daily) with this acupuncture formula, between 66% and 87% (depending on the particular group) obtained good results, that is, symptomatic relief and some reduction in the size of the breast lump.

Behçet's Syndrome

Behçet's syndrome is a rare ulcerative disorder that consists of simultaneous or successive recurrent ulcerations of the oral and genital mucosa, together with uveitis or iridocyclitis. It is often accompanied by arthritis. Other possible manifestations include dermatitis, erythema nodosum, thrombophlebitis, and cerebral involvement. The etiology is probably related to a virus or an immune disorder. Ulcerations tend to be recurrent and are resistant to treatment. Most patients require long-term management by a dermatologist. Cortisone, other immunosuppressants, or immunopotentiators may provide temporary relief but do cause side effects. Unlike the other problems noted in this book, this syndrome also occurs in men, actually with more frequency than in women.

Traditional Chinese medicine views Behçet's syndrome as a "cold ulcer" or a "yin ulcer." Based on the symptoms, it can be differentiated into two types. The first is Kidney and Spleen deficiency: local ulcer, leukorrhea, intolerance of cold, and a purple tongue, which indicates cold and blood stasis. The second type is Kidney yin deficiency: vulvar and ocular itching, pain in the mouth or tongue, and irritability, which indicates Liver fire.

Behçet's Formula 1

STRATEGY: Tonify the Spleen and Kidneys, and invigorate the blood.

Radix Lateralis Aconiti Carmichaeli Praeparata *(fu zi)* 10g
Cortex Cinnamomi Cassiae *(rou gui)* 3g
Rhizoma Pinelliae Ternatae *(ban xia)* 10g
Radix Codonopsitis Pilosulae *(dang shen)* 10g
Radix Astragali Membranacei *(huang qi)* 30g
Rhizoma Atractylodis Macrocephalae *(bai zhu)*.......................10g
Rhizoma Zingiberis Officinalis *(gan jiang)*...............................6g
Sclerotium Poriae Cocos *(fu ling)*..10g
Rhizoma Sparganii Stoloniferi *(san leng)* 10g
Rhizoma Curcumae Ezhu *(e zhu)*..10g
Radix Angelicae Sinensis *(dang gui)*......................................10g

Radix Paeoniae Rubrae *(chi shao)* 10g

Flos Carthami Tinctorii *(hong hua)* 10g

Radix Glycyrrhizae Uralensis *(gan cao)* 3g

METHOD: Take daily as a decoction.

ANALYSIS OF FORMULA: Radix Lateralis Aconiti Carmichaeli Praeparata *(fu zi)* strongly tonifies the Kidneys and Spleen and expels cold. Both Radix Lateralis Aconiti Carmichaeli Praeparata *(fu zi)* and Cortex Cinnamomi Cassiae *(rou gui)* are hot in nature; the former warms the Kidneys, and the latter enters the channels, promotes the circulation of blood, causes sweating, benefits the joints, and relieves angina pectoris (among other actions). It is chosen here primarily to increase local circulation. Rhizoma Zingiberis Officinalis *(gan jiang)* tonifies the Spleen and the Stomach and assists Radix Lateralis Aconiti Carmichaeli Praeparata *(fu zi)* in expelling the cold. Rhizoma Pinelliae Ternatae *(ban xia)*, Rhizoma Atractylodis Macrocephalae *(bai zhu)*, and Sclerotium Poriae Cocos *(fu ling)* remove dampness. Radix Codonopsitis Pilosulae *(dang shen)*, Radix Astragali Membranacei *(huang qi)*, Rhizoma Atractylodis Macrocephalae *(bai zhu)*, and Radix Glycyrrhizae Uralensis *(gan cao)* tonify and help circulate the qi. Rhizoma Curcumae Ezhu *(e zhu)* and Rhizoma Sparganii Stoloniferi *(san leng)*, used together, help the flow of "blood within the qi" as well as the flow of "qi within the blood." Flos Carthami Tinctorii *(hong hua)*, Radix Paeoniae Rubrae *(chi shao)*, and Radix Angelicae Sinensis *(dang gui)* invigorate the blood.

MECHANISM OF ACTION: Radix Lateralis Aconiti Carmichaeli Praeparata *(fu zi)* acts on the adrenal axis and decreases the peripheral eosinocyte count. This function is enhanced when Cortex Cinnamomi Cassiae *(rou gui)* and Rhizoma Zingiberis Officinalis *(gan jiang)* are added to the formula, and suggests that the formula acts by regulating the immune system.

EFFICACY: In one study in which 35 patients with Behçet's syndrome were treated with this formula, five were cured, 19 showed marked improvement, ten were somewhat improved, and one had no improvement.

Behçet's Formula 2

STRATEGY: Replenish the Kidneys, and harmonize the yin and the yang.

Radix Rehmanniae Glutinosae Conquitae *(shu di huang)* 30g
Fructus Corni Officinalis *(shan zhu yu)* 10g
Radix Dioscoreae Oppositae *(shan yao)* 10g
Rhizoma Alismatis Orientalis *(ze xie)* 10g
Sclerotium Poriae Cocos *(fu ling)* 10g
Cortex Moutan Radicis *(mu dan pi)* 10g
Tuber Ophiopogonis Japonici *(mai men dong)* 10g
Radix Paeoniae Lactiflorae *(bai shao)* 10g
Semen Cuscutae Chinensis *(tu si zi)* 10g
Fructus Ligustri Lucidi *(nu zhen zi)* 10g
Fructus Lycii *(gou qi zi)* 10g
Radix Angelicae Sinensis *(dang gui)* 10g
Flos Chrysanthemi Morifolii *(ju hua)* 10g

METHOD: Take daily as a decoction.

ANALYSIS OF FORMULA: Radix Rehmanniae Glutinosae Conquitae *(shu di huang)* replenishes the Kidney yin. Rhizoma Alismatis Orientalis *(ze xie)* drains water from the Kidney channel to mitigate the thick, cloying properties of the former herb. Radix Dioscoreae Oppositae *(shan yao)* strengthens the Spleen yin (that is, its structural aspect, which is the basis for its yang function). Sclerotium Poriae Cocos *(fu ling)* enters the Spleen channel to prevent Radix Dioscoreae Oppositae *(shan yao)* from causing stagnancy. Fructus Corni Officinalis *(shan zhu yu)* and Fructus Ligustri Lucidi *(nu zhen zi)* replenish the Liver and Kidney yin. Cortex Moutan Radicis *(mu dan pi)* quells Liver fire; its relative dryness mitigates the sticky nature of Fructus Corni Officinalis *(shan zhu yu)*. Tuber Ophiopogonis Japonici *(mai men dong)* nourishes the Lung yin. It is used here because the health of the Lungs affects the skin. Radix Angelicae Sinensis *(dang gui)* tonifies the blood. Flos Chrysanthemi Morifolii *(ju hua)* clears fire from the Liver and benefits the eyes. This formula is well-organized to harmonize the functions of the Kidneys, Spleen, and Liver, especially when yin deficiency results in Liver fire.

EFFICACY: In one study in which 28 patients with Behçet's syndrome were treated with the above formula, seven were cured, nine showed marked improvement, ten showed some improvement, and two had no improvement.

Acne

Acne usually occurs at puberty when the sebaceous glands, stimulated by androgens, mature and accumulate sebum. When the sebum reaches the surface of the skin, it comes into contact with bacteria and the gland can become a site of infection. Acne can present as open or closed comedones (infected hair follicles) or as pustules, mostly on the face, chest, and back. Topical treatment such as lotion, soap, or astringents may be used. Estrogen and vitamins are also suggested. If the infection is deep or severe, antibiotics may be prescribed.

According to traditional Chinese medicine, the skin is linked with the Lungs, while the face, mouth, and lips are associated with the Spleen. Acne is thus seen as a disorder of the Lungs and Spleen. During puberty, while the Kidneys are flourishing, heat may rise up to the Lungs and Stomach, causing heat in both of these Organs.

Acne Formula 1

STRATEGY: Remove excessive heat from the Lungs and Stomach.

Folium Eriobotryae Japonicae *(pi pa ye)* 9g
Cortex Mori Albae Radicis *(sang bai pi)* 9g
Rhizoma Coptidis *(huang lian)* 6g
Cortex Phellodendri *(huang bai)* 9g
Radix Glycyrrhizae Uralensis *(gan cao)* 6g
Radix Ginseng *(ren shen)* 6g

METHOD: Take daily as a decoction.

MODIFICATIONS:

1. If there is intense Stomach heat (tender red pustules, thirst, dark urine, constipation, and a red tongue with a yellow coating), omit Radix Ginseng *(ren shen),* and add:
Gypsum*(shi gao)* 9g
Cooked Radix et Rhizoma Rhei *(zhi da huang)* 9g
Radix Arnebiae seu Lithospermi *(zi cao)* 12g
Fructus Sophorae Japonicae Immaturus *(huai hua mi)* 12g

2. If there is blood stasis (dark face, thirst, dark tongue), omit Radix Ginseng *(ren shen),* and add:
Flos Carthami Tinctorii *(hong hua)* 6g
Hirudo seu Whitmaniae *(shui zhi)* 6g
Spina Gleditsiae Sinensis *(zao jiao ci)* 12g
Semen Vaccariae Segetalis *(wang bu liu xing)* 12g

3. If there is dampness (exudation, poor appetite, abdominal distention, white tongue coating), omit Radix Ginseng *(ren shen),* and add:
Semen Coicis Lachryma-jobi *(yi yi ren)* 12g
Radix Sophorae Flavescentis *(ku shen)* 9g
Rhizoma Smilacis Glabrae *(tu fu ling)* 15g

ANALYSIS OF FORMULA: Folium Eriobotryae Japonicae *(pi pa ye)* and Cortex Mori Albae Radicis *(sang bai pi)* expel heat from the Lungs. Rhizoma Coptidis *(huang lian),* Cortex Phellodendri *(huang bai),* and Gypsum*(shi gao)* purge the heat from the Stomach, and cooked Radix et Rhizoma Rhei *(zhi da huang)* removes the heat downward through the bowels, which also helps purge the heat from the Lungs. Radix Arnebiae seu Lithospermi *(zi cao)* and Fructus Sophorae Japonicae Immaturus *(huai hua mi)* clear heat. Semen Coicis Lachryma-jobi *(yi yi ren),* Radix Sophorae Flavescentis *(ku shen),* and Rhizoma Smilacis Glabrae *(tu fu ling)* clear heat and drain dampness. Flos Carthami Tinctorii *(hong hua)* and Hirudo seu Whitmaniae *(shui zhi)* remove blood stasis. Spina Gleditsiae Sinensis *(zao jiao ci)* and Semen Vaccariae Segetalis *(wang bu* *liu xing)* promote the flow of qi. Radix Ginseng *(ren shen)* and Radix Glycyrrhizae Uralensis *(gan cao)* tonify the qi in order to facilitate its flow.

MECHANISM OF ACTION: The mechanism of action has yet to be identified.

EFFICACY: In a study of 103 adolescent patients treated with this formula (and without antibiotics), 90 experienced a complete resolution of symptoms, eight improved, and five showed no improvement and required antibiotics. Results were similar for males and females.

Acne Formula 2

STRATEGY: Replenish the Kidneys, Spleen, and Lungs.

Herba Epimedii *(yin yang huo)* 15g
Rhizoma Polygonati *(huang jing)* 15g
Rhizoma Polygonati Odorati *(yu zhu)* 15g

METHOD: Take daily as a decoction.

ANALYSIS OF FORMULA: Herba Epimedii *(yin yang huo)* replenishes the yin and the yang of the Kidneys. Rhizoma Polygonati *(huang jing)* and Rhizoma Polygonati Odorati *(yu zhu)* tonify the Lungs and the Spleen and thus reduce heat.

MECHANISM OF ACTION: This formula is directed at the root cause of acne, namely the Lungs, Spleen, and Kidneys. It works by increasing serum E_2 levels while decreasing T levels. SHBG values are unchanged. Blood HDL levels are increased and triglycerides are decreased. This suggests an action on the endocrine and metabolic systems.

EFFICACY: In a study of 30 adolescent patients treated with this formula (and without antibiotics), 24 had a complete resolution of symptoms, while six improved but relapsed when treatment was stopped. Results were similar for males and females.

Endometriosis and Adenomyosis

Endometriosis consists of the presence of functional endometrium outside of the uterus. Common symptoms are dysmenorrhea, infertility, and pelvic pain. Most of the implants bleed into the peritoneal cavity during menstruation, which produces chemical irritation and adhesions. An inflammatory pseudocapsule over the ovaries may interfere with their function. Adenomyosis is the benign invasion of the endometrium into the myometrium. The uterus is enlarged. Dysmenorrhea and abnormal bleeding may be caused by the increased vascularity. Myometrial contractility may be increased by the presence of ectopic endometrium. Both diseases therefore have similar symptoms, and adenomyosis is present in 15% of patients with endometriosis. Various treatments can be considered depending on the patient's condition. Analgesics, hormonal therapy, or conservative surgery afford temporary relief and can be considered for young patients, to remedy infertility, or in mild or moderate cases. Oophorectomy and total hysterectomy give good results if the patient is willing to sacrifice ovarian and reproductive functions.

Traditional Chinese medicine views both conditions as "dysmenorrhea" and "mass in the Womb." When the endometrium implants itself on the bronchial or nasal mucosa, it is called "vicarious menstruation." (This condition probably results from endometrial tissue being carried in the blood stream.) Fever caused by chemical irritation due to intraperitoneal bleeding is called "menstrual fever." All of these conditions are seen as the result of blood stasis in the Lower Burner, which may be accompanied by yin deficiency and Lung heat or Liver fire.

Endometriosis Formula 1

STRATEGY: Invigorate the blood and dispel blood stasis.

Radix Bupleuri *(chai hu)* 9g
Radix Angelicae Sinensis *(dang gui)* 9g
Pollen Typhae *(pu huang)* 12g
Excrementum Trogopterori seu Pteromi *(wu ling zhi)* 12g

Rhizoma Sparganii Stoloniferi *(san leng)*................................9g

Rhizoma Curcumae Ezhu *(e zhu)*................................9g

Rhizoma Cyperi Rotundi *(xiang fu)*................................9g

Rhizoma Corydalis Yanhusuo *(yan hu suo)*................................5g

Herba cum Radix Cynanchi Paniculati *(xu chang qing)*................15g

Spina Gleditsiae Sinensis *(zao jiao ci)*................................9g

Eupolyphaga seu Opisthoplatia *(tu bie chong)*........................12g

METHOD: Take daily as a decoction.

MODIFICATIONS:

1. With qi deficiency, omit Radix Bupleuri *(chai hu)* and Rhizoma Cyperi Rotundi *(xiang fu)*, and add:

    Radix Codonopsitis Pilosulae *(dang shen)*............................12g

    Radix Astragali Membranacei *(huang qi)*............................12g

    Rhizoma Cimicifugae *(sheng ma)*................................9g

2. With intolerance to cold, add:

    Ramulus Cinnamomi Cassiae *(gui zhi)*................................6g

3. With constipation, add:

    Cooked Radix et Rhizoma Rhei *(zhi da huang)*........................6g

4. With premenstrual pain, add:

    Radix Rubiae Cordifoliae *(qian cao gen)*............................15g

    Fructus Sophorae Japonicae Immaturus *(huai hua mi)*...............15g

ANALYSIS OF FORMULA: Radix Bupleuri *(chai hu)*, Rhizoma Cyperi Rotundi *(xiang fu)*, Rhizoma Corydalis Yanhusuo *(yan hu suo)*, and Herba cum Radix Cynanchi Paniculati *(xu chang qing)* promote the flow of Liver qi and thereby relieve pain. Pollen Typhae *(pu huang)*, Excrementum Trogopterori seu Pteromi *(wu ling zhi)*, Rhizoma Sparganii Stoloniferi *(san leng)*, Rhizoma Curcumae Ezhu *(e zhu)*, and Eupolyphaga seu Opisthoplatia *(tu bie chong)* are selected to invigorate the blood, remove blood stasis, relieve pain, and dissolve congealed blood. Ramulus Cinnamomi

Cassiae *(gui zhi)* warms and clears the channels. Cooked Radix et Rhizoma Rhei *(zhi da huang)* invigorates the blood and expels heat.

MECHANISM OF ACTION: This formula reduces blood viscosity. There is a proven relationship between high blood viscosity and abnormal prostaglandin levels. In general, herbs that invigorate the blood do so by reducing blood viscosity, and by regulating the level of prostaglandins.

EFFICACY: In one study, treatment was given for six to 12 months to 156 patients with various presentations of endometriosis and adenomyosis. Eighty-nine patients experienced significant relief of pain, menstrual disorders, and other symptoms. Thirty-nine patients showed some improvement, while 28 had no result or relapsed.

Endometriosis Formula 2

This is actually a group of three prescriptions. The first is to be taken for five to seven days before the menses, the second during menstruation, and the third for the other days in the cycle.

• Formula to use just before menstruation

STRATEGY: Relieve the stagnancy of qi and blood.

Pollen Typhae *(pu huang)* 12g
Excrementum Trogopterori seu Pteromi *(wu ling zhi)* 12g
Radix Salviae Miltiorrhizae *(dan shen)* 12g
Radix Achyranthis Bidentatae *(niu xi)* 12g
Gummi Olibanum *(ru xiang)* 3g
Myrrha *(mo yao)* 3g
Rhizoma Sparganii Stoloniferi *(san leng)* 9g
Rhizoma Curcumae Ezhu *(e zhu)* 9g
Herba Artemisiae Anomalae *(liu ji nu)* 15g
Radix Notoginseng *(san qi)* 0.4g

• Formula to use during menstruation

STRATEGY: Dispel blood stasis to control menstruation.

Pollen Typhae *(pu huang)* 12g
Excrementum Trogopterori seu Pteromi *(wu ling zhi)* 12g
Ophicalcitum *(hua rui shi)* 30g
Rhizoma Cyperi Rotundi *(xiang fu)* 9g
Radix Linderae Strychnifoliae *(wu yao)* 9g
Radix Ligustici Chuanxiong *(chuan xiong)* 6g
Cooked Radix et Rhizoma Rhei *(zhi da huang)* 6g
Radix Astragali Membranacei *(huang qi)* 15g
Cortex Cinnamomi Cassiae *(rou gui)* 3g

• Formula to use during the other days of the cycle

STRATEGY: Soften and break up masses, dispel blood stasis, and tonify the
Kidneys.

Ramulus Cinnamomi Cassiae *(gui zhi)* 9g
Radix Paeoniae Rubrae *(chi shao)* 12g
Cortex Moutan Radicis *(mu dan pi)* 12g
Semen Persicae *(tao ren)* 9g
Thallus Algae *(kun bu)* 12g
Rhizoma Sparganii Stoloniferi *(san leng)* 12g
Rhizoma Curcumae Ezhu *(e zhu)* 12g
Carapax Amydae Sinensis *(bie jia)* 15g
Sclerotium Poriae Cocos *(fu ling)* 15g
Herba Cynomorii Songarici *(suo yang)* 15g
Herba Epimedii *(yin yang huo)* 30g
Eupolyphaga seu Opisthoplatia *(tu bie chong)* 15g
Semen Vaccariae Segetalis *(wang bu liu xing)* 12g

ANALYSIS OF FORMULAS: Radix Paeoniae Rubrae *(chi shao)*, Cortex
Moutan Radicis *(mu dan pi)*, Semen Persicae *(tao ren)*, Rhizoma Cyperi

Rotundi *(xiang fu)*, Radix Linderae Strychnifoliae *(wu yao)*, Rhizoma Sparganii Stoloniferi *(san leng)*, Rhizoma Curcumae Ezhu *(e zhu)*, and Semen Vaccariae Segetalis *(wang bu liu xing)* together promote the flow of qi and blood, dispel blood stasis, and relieve pain. Pollen Typhae *(pu huang)*, Excrementum Trogopterori seu Pteromi *(wu ling zhi)*, Ophicalcitum *(hua rui shi)*, Gummi Olibanum *(ru xiang)*, Myrrha*(mo yao)*, Radix Notoginseng *(san qi)*, and Herba Artemisiae Anomalae *(liu ji nu)* dispel blood stasis and stop bleeding. In general, bleeding due to stasis is increased in endometriosis and adenomyosis, which is why herbs are included in this formula to stop bleeding. Carapax Amydae Sinensis *(bie jia)*, Thallus Algae *(kun bu)*, Rhizoma Sparganii Stoloniferi *(san leng)*, Rhizoma Curcumae Ezhu *(e zhu)*, and Eupolyphaga seu Opisthoplatia *(tu bie chong)* break up masses and promote the flow of qi and blood. Endometriosis and adenomyosis are often accompanied by anovulation due to interference from prostaglandins and the immune system. Thus Herba Cynomorii Songarici *(suo yang)* and Herba Epimedii *(yin yang huo)* are used in this formula to tonify the Kidneys and improve ovarian function. Radix Astragali Membranacei *(huang qi)* and Ramulus Cinnamomi Cassiae *(gui zhi)* augment and warm the qi. Cooked Radix et Rhizoma Rhei *(zhi da huang)* removes blood stasis and expels the heat associated with it.

MECHANISM OF ACTION: When used consistently, this formula helps reduce blood viscosity.

EFFICACY: In a study of 60 patients with endometriosis and adenomyosis who were treated for six to 12 months with this formula, 29 experienced symptomatic relief or reduction in the size of the mass, or became pregnant (when they had originally consulted for infertility). Eighteen obtained some improvement in their symptoms, 11 improved but relapsed, and two had no improvement.

Endometriosis Formula 3

STRATEGY: Replenish the yin in order to subdue the fire, and redirect the upward flow of blood (as in vicarious menstruation) downward.

Radix Rehmanniae Glutinosae *(sheng di huang)* 15g

Radix Scrophulariae Ningpoensis *(xuan shen)* 12g

Fructus Lycii *(gou qi zi)* 12g

Cortex Moutan Radicis *(mu dan pi)* 6g

Radix Salviae Miltiorrhizae *(dan shen)*................................12g

Rhizoma Polygonati Odorati *(yu zhu)*...................................12g

Fructus Gardeniae Jasminoidis *(zhi zi)*...............................12g

Radix Achyranthis Bidentatae *(niu xi)*.................................9g

Radix Rubiae Cordifoliae *(qian cao gen)*..............................12g

Tuber Curcumae *(yu jin)*..9g

METHOD: Take daily as a decoction.

ANALYSIS OF FORMULA: Radix Rehmanniae Glutinosae *(sheng di huang)*, Fructus Lycii *(gou qi zi)*, Radix Scrophulariae Ningpoensis *(xuan shen)*, and Rhizoma Polygonati Odorati *(yu zhu)* tonify the yin of the Lungs, Liver, and Kidneys. Radix Scrophulariae Ningpoensis *(xuan shen)*, Cortex Moutan Radicis *(mu dan pi)*, Fructus Gardeniae Jasminoidis *(zhi zi)*, and Tuber Curcumae *(yu jin)* clear heat from the Lungs and the Liver. Radix Achyranthis Bidentatae *(niu xi)* redirects the flow of blood downward. Radix Rubiae Cordifoliae *(qian cao gen)* dispels blood stasis in order to stop the bleeding.

MECHANISM OF ACTION: The mechanism of action has yet to be identified.

EFFICACY: In a study of 21 patients with menstrual hemoptysis treated with the above formula for three to five months, 20 were cured and one showed little if any result.

Endometriosis Formula 4

STRATEGY: Subdue the fire and dispel blood stasis to relieve the menstrual fever.

Rhizoma Anemarrhenae Asphodeloidis *(zhi mu)* 12g

Gypsum *(shi gao)*... 9g

Herba Artemisiae Annuae *(qing hao)* 12g

Cortex Moutan Radicis *(mu dan pi)*.................................... 12g

Fructus Gardeniae Jasminoidis *(zhi zi)*................................. 12g

Carapax Amydae Sinensis *(bie jia)* 12g

Radix Rehmanniae Glutinosae *(sheng di huang)* 12g

Radix Salviae Miltiorrhizae *(dan shen)*................................ 12g

Pollen Typhae *(pu huang)* 12g

Excrementum Trogopterori seu Pteromi *(wu ling zhi)*............ 12g

Semen Persicae *(tao ren)* 12g

Fructus Meliae Toosendan *(chuan lian zi)* 12g

Herba Artemisiae Anomalae *(liu ji nu)*................................. 12g

METHOD: Take daily as a decoction.

ANALYSIS OF FORMULA: Rhizoma Anemarrhenae Asphodeloidis *(zhi mu)* and Gypsum *(shi gao)* clear heat from the blood. Herba Artemisiae Annuae *(qing hao)*, Cortex Moutan Radicis *(mu dan pi)*, and Fructus Gardeniae Jasminoidis *(zhi zi)* clear Liver heat. Radix Rehmanniae Glutinosae *(sheng di huang)* and Carapax Amydae Sinensis *(bie jia)* replenish the yin. Radix Salviae Miltiorrhizae *(dan shen)*, Pollen Typhae *(pu huang)*, Excrementum Trogopterori seu Pteromi *(wu ling zhi)*, Herba Artemisiae Anomalae *(liu ji nu)*, and Semen Persicae *(tao ren)* dispel blood stasis. Fructus Meliae Toosendan *(chuan lian zi)* regulates the qi of the Liver.

MECHANISM OF ACTION: The mechanism of action has yet to be determined.

EFFICACY: Good results have been obtained with this formula in abating the fever associated with endometriosis. In one study of 12 patients with endometriosis and menstrual fever, the fever subsided within two cycles without relapse.

Supplemental Materia Medica

This appendix contains descriptions of materia medica found in this text but which are not listed in *Chinese Herbal Medicine: Materia Medica*, by Bensky and Gamble. Since readers may not be familiar with these medicinal substances, we present basic information about them here in an abbreviated version of the format used in that book. They are arranged in alphbetical order based on their *pīnyīn* name.

lù xián cǎo
鹿衔草

PHARMACEUTICAL NAME: Herba Pyrolae Rotundifoliae
BOTANICAL NAME: *Pyrola rotundifolia* L.
FAMILY: pyrolaceae
ALTERNATE NAMES: 鹿含草 *lù hán cǎo*
ENGLISH: Pyrola
LITERAL ENGLISH TRANSLATION: "deer bit herb"
PROPERTIES: sweet, bitter, warm
CHANNELS ENTERED: Liver, Kidneys

ACTIONS AND INDICATIONS:

- Dispels wind-dampness and strengthens the sinews and bones: for wind-damp painful obstruction and weakness of the sinews and bones. Often used in the elderly. Also used for bone spurs.
- Tonifies the Kidneys and moistens the Lungs: for lower back pain accompanied by cold, painful feet from Kidney deficiency. Also for chronic cough from Lung deficiency, chronic dryness, or Kidneys not grasping the Qi.
- Stops bleeding: for various types of bleeding, including nosebleed, vomiting blood, and excessive menstruation.
- Nourishes the Heart and restrains sweating: for palpitiations with night sweats.

CAUTIONS AND CONTRAINDICATIONS: None noted

DOSAGE: 15-30g.

nán guā dì

南瓜蒂

PHARMACEUTICAL NAME: Pedicellus Cucurbitae Moschatae

BOTANICAL NAME: *Cucurbita moschata* Duch.

FAMILY: cucurbitaceae

ENGLISH: pumpkin pedicle

LITERAL ENGLISH TRANSLATION: "southern melon pedicle"

PROPERTIES: bitter, cold

CHANNELS ENTERED: Lung, Liver

ACTIONS AND INDICATIONS:

- Relieves toxicity and reduces swelling: for any swelling with toxiciy such as abscesses or burns.
- Clears heat, strenghtens the Womb, and calms the fetus: for pathogenic heat disturbing the Womb with a restless fetus.

CAUTIONS AND CONTRAINDICATIONS: None noted.

DOSAGE: 9-30g. Used externally as a powder.

shēn jīn cǎo

伸筋草

PHARMACEUTICAL NAME: Herba cum Radice Lycopodii Clavati

BOTANICAL NAME: *Lycopodium clavatum* L. In some parts of China, *Smilax nipponica* Miq. is used as this herb.

FAMILY: lycopodiaceae

ENGLISH: running pine, staghorn clubmoss

LITERAL ENGLISH TRANSLATION: "extend sinew herb"

PROPERTIES: bitter, acrid, warm

CHANNELS ENTERED: Liver, Spleen, Kidney

ACTIONS AND INDICATIONS:

• Dispels wind and scatters cold, eliminates dampness and swelling, relaxes the sinews, and invigorates the collaterals: for painful obstruction due to wind, cold, and dampness, especially of the joints; numbness of the skin; weakness of the extremities; trauma and contusions

CAUTIONS AND CONTRAINDICATIONS: Contraindicated during pregnancy and in cases of hemorrhaging.

DOSAGE: 9-15 g.

tiān xiān téng

天仙藤

PHARMACEUTICAL NAME: Caulis Aristolochiae

BOTANICAL NAME: *Aristolochia debilis* Sieb. et Zucc. or *A. contorta* Bge.

FAMILY: aristolochaceae

ALTERNATE NAMES: 马兜铃藤 *mǎ dōu líng téng*

ENGLISH: birthwort caulis, aristolochia caulis

LITERAL ENGLISH TRANSLATION: "heavenly immortal caulis"

PROPERTIES: bitter, warm

CHANNELS ENTERED: Liver, Spleen, Kidneys

ACTIONS AND INDICATIONS:

• Dispels wind and resolves dampness: for pain from wind-dampness and edema during pregnancy.

• Invigorates the blood and stops pain: for pain in the chest, epigastrium, or abdomen. Often used for postpartum abdominal pain from blood stasis.

CAUTIONS AND CONTRAINDICATIONS: None noted.

DOSAGE: 4.5-9g.

tòu gǔ cǎo
透骨草

PHARMACEUTICAL NAME: Herba Speranskiae seu Impatientis

BOTANICAL NAME: *Speranskia tuberculata* (Bge.) Baill. or *Impatiens balsamina* L.

Families: euphorbiaceae

ENGLISH: speranskia or balsam

LITERAL ENGLISH TRANSLATION: "penetrate bone grass"

PROPERTIES: sweet, acrid, warm

CHANNELS ENTERED: Lung, Liver

ACTIONS AND INDICATIONS:

- Dispels wind and eliminates dampness: for painful obstruction due to wind-dampness, leg-qi due to cold-dampness; also for the inward sinking of toxin from sores and tinea.
- Relaxes the sinews and invigorates the collaterals: for muscular contractions and tension or spasms.
- Inviogrates the blood and stops pain: for pain anywhere in the body, including the trunk and limbs.
- Relieves toxicity and transforms rashes: for rashes due to heat or toxic swellings including those of the extrernal genitalia.

CAUTIONS AND CONTRAINDICATIONS: Contraindicated during pregnancy.

DOSAGE: 9-15 g.

xú cháng qīng
徐长卿

PHARMACEUTICAL NAME: Herba cum Radix Cynanchi Paniculati

BOTANICAL NAME: *Cynanchum paniculatum* (Bge.) Kitag.

FAMILY: asclepiadaceae

ALTERNATE NAMES: 寮刁竹 *liáo diāo zhú*

ENGLISH: cynanchum paniculatum

LITERAL ENGLISH TRANSLATION: "slow long-lasting minister"

PROPERTIES: acrid, warm

CHANNELS ENTERED: Liver, Stomach

ACTIONS AND INDICATIONS:

- Dispels wind and stops pain: for pain including wind-damp painful obstruction, pain from trauma, abdominal pain, or toothache. As this herb

has a reltively good effect at dispelling wind and stopping pain, it can be used for pain from wind-dampness, cold congealing, qi stagnation, or blood stasis. Recently used for postoperative pain and the pain accompanying tumors.
- Dispels wind and stops itching: for skin problems such as eczema, urticaria, or stubborn cases of tinea.
- Also used topically for poisonous snake bite.

CAUTIONS AND CONTRAINDICATIONS: Use cautiously in the debilitated.

DOSAGE: 3-10g in decoctions; 1.5-3g in powders. Do not decoct for long as it is aromatic.

xún gǔ fēng
寻骨风

PHARMACEUTICAL NAME: Rhizoma seu Herba Aristolochiae Mollissimae

BOTANICAL NAME: *Aristolochia mollissima* Hance.

FAMILY: aristolochiae

ENGLISH: root or entire plant of hairy birthwort or artistolochia mollissima

LITERAL ENGLISH TRANSLATION: "seek bone wind"

PROPERTIES: acrid, bitter, neutral

CHANNEL ENTERED: Liver

ACTIONS AND INDICATIONS:
- Dispels wind, unblocks the collaterals, and stops pain: for wind-damp painful obstruction with numbness and paresthesia and spasms of the sinews. Also for pain secondary to trauma.
- Also used for stomachace or toothache.

CAUTIONS AND CONTRAINDICATIONS: Some sources state that this herb should not be used when there in internal heat from yin deficiency.

DOSAGE: 9-15g. Can be used in tinctures or linaments.

yā zhí cǎo
鸭跖草

PHARMACEUTICAL NAME: Herba Commelinae Communis

BOTANICAL NAME: *Commelina communis* L.

FAMILY: commelinaceae

ENGLISH: day flower, commelina

LITERAL ENGLISH TRANSLATION: "duck-walk herb"

PROPERTIES: sweet, bitter, cold

CHANNELS ENTERED: Lung, Stomach, Bladder

ACTIONS AND INDICATIONS:

- Clears heat, relieves toxicity, and reduces fever: for fever from either exterior heat or qi level heat.
- Clears heat, promotes urination, and unblocks painful urinary dysfunction: for hot painful urinary dysfunction or edema with heat.
- Clears heat, relieves toxicity, and treats sores: for various sores or swellings due to heat toxicity including, sore throat, sores, abscesses, and snakebite. Can be applied both internally and locally.

CAUTIONS AND CONTRAINDICATIONS: None noted.

DOSAGE: 15-30g; fresh 30-60g; externally as needed.

zhù má gēn

苎麻根

PHARMACEUTICAL NAME: Radix Boehmeriae

BOTANICAL NAME: *Boehmeria nivea* (L.) Gaud.

FAMILY: urticaceae

ENGLISH: ramie root

PROPERTIES: sweet, cold

CHANNELS ENTERED: Heart, Liver

ACTIONS AND INDICATIONS:

- Cools the blood and stops bleeding: for any type of bleeding due to heat, including coughing blood, vomiting blood, uterine bleeding, and thrombocytopenic purpura.
- Clears heat and calms the fetus: for restless fetus or bleeding during pregnancy secondary to a heat collecting during pregnancy.
- Clears heat and promotes urination: for damp-heat in the lower burner and painful urinary dysfunction with dribbling of urine.

CAUTIONS AND CONTRAINDICATIONS: Not to be used for cold conditions.

DOSAGE: 9-30g. Used externally as a powder.

References

The materials used in this book were selected by myself and my colleagues over many years. During this time we did not record full bibliographic information about each of the studies mentioned in the text. However, the primary books and journals that we consulted for this purpose are listed below.

Journals

Acupuncture Research (Zhen ci yan jiu) 针刺研究

Beijing Traditional Chinese Medicine (Beijing zhong yi) 北京中医

Chinese Journal of Acupuncture and Moxibustion (Zhong guo zhen jiu) 中国针灸

Chinese Journal of Integrated Traditional and Western Medicine (Zhong guo zhong xi yi jie he za zhi) 中国中西医结合杂志

Chinese Journal of Obstetrics and Gynecology (Zhong hua fu chan ke za zhi) 中华妇产科杂志

Hubei Journal of Traditional Chinese Medicine (Hubei zhong yi za zhi)
湖北中医杂志

Jiangsu Journal of Traditional Chinese Medicine (Jiangsu zhong yi za zhi)
江苏中医杂志

Journal of Reproductive Medicine (Sheng zhi yi xue za zhi) 生殖医学杂志

Journal of Traditional Chinese Medicine (Zhong yi za zhi) 中医杂志

Shandong Journal of Traditional Chinese Medicine (Shandong zhong yi za zhi) 山东中医杂志

Shanghai Journal of Traditional Chinese Medicine (Shanghai zhong yi yao za zhi) 上海中医药杂志

Zhejiang Journal of Traditional Chinese Medicine (Zhejiang zhong yi za zhi) 浙江中医杂志

Books

Shanghai College of Traditional Chinese Medicine, Faculty of Materia Medica, *Lectures on Chinese Materia Medica (Zhong yao xue jiang yi)* 中药学讲义. Shanghai: Shanghai Science and Technology Press, 1959.

Wu She-Ming, ed., *Collection of Chinese Traditional Secret Formulas (Zhong guo zhong yi mi fang da quan)* 中国中医秘方大全. Shanghai: Wenhui Publishing Company, 1989.

Zhou Jin-Huang, Wang Jia-Zhong, ed., *Advances in Pharmacological and Clinical Studies on Chinese Materia Medica*, volumes 1-4 *(Zhong yao yao li yu lin chuang yan jiu jin zhan)* 中药药理与临床研究进展. Beijing: Military Science Publishing Company, 1992-1996.

Point and Herb Index

D

E

F

N

O

P

T

General Index